Respiratory Medicine

To Sir John Crofton,
Professor Emeritus of Respiratory Diseases,
University of Edinburgh

and

To Dr Andrew Douglas,
Reader in Respiratory Medicine,
University of Edinburgh

Respiratory Medicine

FIRST EDITION BY

Malcolm Schonell

MB, BS (Qld), MD (NSW), FCCP, FRCP (Edin.), FRACP
Consultant Respiratory Physician, St George Hospital, Sydney. Formerly Associate
Professor of Medicine, University of New South Wales, Australia.

REVISED BY

Ian Campbell

BSc, MB, BS, MD (Lond.), FRCP (Edin.)
Consultant in Thoracic Medicine, Llandough and Sully Hospitals, Cardiff, Wales.

SECOND EDITION

CHURCHILL LIVINGSTONE
EDINBURGH LONDON MELBOURNE AND NEW YORK 1984

CHURCHILL LIVINGSTONE
Medical Division of Longman Group Limited

Distributed in the United States of America by
Churchill Livingstone Inc., 1560 Broadway, New York,
N.Y. 10036, and by associated companies, branches and
representatives throughout the world.

First Edition 1974
Second Edition 1984

ISBN 0 443 01834 0

British Library Cataloguing in Publication Data
Schonell, Malcolm
    Respiratory medicine.—2nd ed.
    1. Respiratory organs—Diseases
    I. Title   II. Campbell, Ian
    616.2   RC731

Library of Congress Cataloging in Publication Data
Schonell, Malcolm.
    Respiratory medicine.
    Includes index.
    1. Respiratory organs—Diseases. I. Campbell,
Ian, M.D.   II. Title.   [DNLM: 1. Respiratory tract
diseases.   WF 140 S371r]
RC731.S3   1984   616.2   83-15177

Printed in Singapore by Selector Printing Co (Pte) Ltd

Preface to Second Edition

Since 1974 there have been changes in respiratory medicine. It has been a pleasure to revise Malcolm Schonell's excellent textbook to incorporate the advances of recent years.

My special thanks are due to Mrs Elizabeth Lyons for typing the manuscript and to Anne, Colin, Sarah and Andrew for their tolerance.

1984   I.A.C.

Preface to the First Edition

My main aim in writing this small book has been to present a practical and lucid approach to respiratory medicine. While the book is intended primarily for students I hope that it will be helpful to those studying for postgraduate qualifications and to doctors confronted with a clinical problem.

I wish to thank my students, my Senior Registrar, Dr J. R. Govan, Dr A. C. Douglas, Associate Professor B. H. Gandevia, Mr D. A. Horton, Dr G. J. R. McHardy and Professor W. R. Pitney for helpful comments on individual chapters. Dr N. W. Horne read the complete manuscript and I am most grateful for his authoritative opinion. While acknowledging the advice of my colleagues I accept responsibility for the final text.

My special thanks are due to Mrs C. J. Joyce and Mrs N. M. Conlon for graciously typing many drafts of the manuscript and to Miss J. Crossley, Miss C. de Lambert and to my wife, Margaret, for preparing the illustrations.

It is a pleasure to acknowledge the assistance of the staff of Churchill Livingstone.

My wife and children gave me continued encouragement during my seemingly endless task and for this I am especially appreciative.

1974   MALCOLM SCHONELL

Contents

Contents

1

Structure and function of the respiratory system

The respiratory system may be divided into the upper and lower respiratory tracts. The lower respiratory tract lies below the cricoid cartilage and includes the trachea, bronchi, lungs and pleura. The upper and lower respiratory tracts are related in structure and function, and disease of one may affect the other. Respiratory medicine is concerned with diseases which predominantly affect the lower respiratory tract.

Upper respiratory tract

This comprises the nose, nasal sinuses, nasopharynx and larynx. The upper respiratory tract warms and humidifies the inspired air and is lined by mucus secreting ciliated columnar epithelium which acts as a protective barrier. Bacteria and particulate matter are trapped by the mucus which is propelled upwards by cilial action and is then expectorated. The epiglottic or gag reflex and the cough reflex prevent inhalation of large particles of foreign material.

Cough reflex

This is a vital defence mechanism which is initiated by the presence of irritant gas, foreign material or excessive secretions in the larynx, trachea or bronchi. Diseases of the respiratory tract commonly cause cough. A cough consists of three phases: a deep inspiration, forced expiration against a closed glottis and an explosive expiratory blast due to sudden opening of the vocal cords. Impairment of the cough reflex predisposes to inhalation of foreign material. This may occur during anaesthesia or after drug overdose or alcohol intoxication and may cause pneumonia or lung abscess.

The main motor nerve to the larynx is the recurrent laryngeal nerve, which is a branch of the vagus. On the left side the recurrent laryngeal nerve arises from the vagus near the hilum of the left lung and after passing under the aortic arch runs upwards to the larynx. Bronchial carcinoma in the region of the left hilum may involve the recurrent laryngeal nerve causing hoarseness due to paralysis of the left vocal cord.

Trachea and bronchi

The trachea begins at the lower border of the cricoid cartilage and ends at the level of the sternal angle where it bifurcates into the right and left main bronchi. The spur of cartilage between the two main bronchi is called the main carina. The right main bronchus follows the line of the trachea more closely than the left main bronchus, and for this reason inhaled foreign material is more likely to enter the right lung than the left.

The right main bronchus gives rise to three lobar bronchi. About 2 cm from the main carina the right upper lobe bronchus arises from the lateral wall of the main bronchus at an angle of 90°. The middle lobe bronchus then arises from the anterior wall, after which the downward continuation of the main bronchus becomes the lower lobe bronchus.

The left main bronchus gives rise to two lobar bronchi. The upper lobe bronchus arises from the lateral wall about 5 cm from the main carina; the main bronchus then becomes the lower lobe bronchus.

The lobar bronchi each divide into two or more segmental bronchi (Fig. 1).

The lingular bronchus which runs downwards from the left upper lobe bronchus supplies a segment of lung on the left side, the lingula, which corresponds to the middle lobe on the right. The bronchus to the apical segment of each lower lobe arises from the posterior wall of the lower lobe bronchus. There is no medial basal segment in the left lower lobe. The main bronchi, lobar bronchi and the orifices of the segmental bronchi can be seen readily on bronchoscopy (p. 53). Knowledge of the segmental anatomy explains why inhaled foreign material is more likely to lodge in certain segments of the lung than others (p. 94).

The trachea and bronchi are composed of mucosa, submucosa and a fibro-cartilaginous layer containing plain muscle. The mucosa is lined with ciliated columnar epithelium and contains mucus secreting goblet cells. Mucous glands are present in the submucosa. The trachea and main bronchi are supported on their anterior and lateral aspects by horseshoe shaped plates of cartilage and the posterior deficiency is supported by muscle fibres. Cartilage is irregularly distributed in the walls of the lobar bronchi where they enter the lung substance and in the walls of the segmental and smaller bronchi.

Interlobar fissures

The surface markings of the interlobar fissures delineate the position of the lobes of the lungs, and abnormalities detected on physical examination are described in relation to their lobar distribution. The

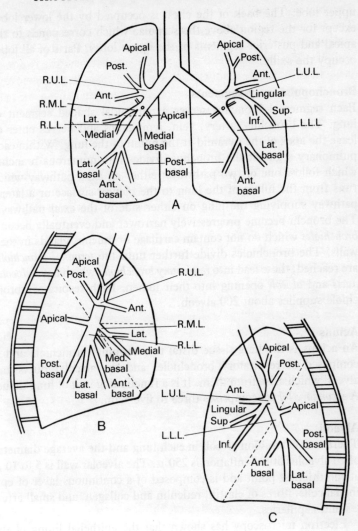

Fig. 1 The anatomy of the tracheobronchial tree. (A) Anterior view; (B) Right lung, lateral view; (C) Left lung, lateral view.

oblique fissure is indicated by a curved line drawn from the 2nd thoracic spine to the 6th rib in the mid-clavicular line. On the right side, the horizontal fissure is marked by a line drawn from the sternum at the level of the 4th costal cartilage to meet the oblique fissure in the axilla. The front of the chest above the horizontal fissure corresponds to the upper lobe and below the fissure to the right middle lobe. On the left, the front of the chest is mainly occupied by the upper lobe. The back of the chest is occupied by the lower lobes except for the region above the scapulae which corresponds to the apical and posterior segments of the upper lobes. Parts of all lobes occupy the axilla.

Bronchopulmonary segments

Each segmental bronchus serves a pyramidal shaped segment of lung. The bronchus, artery, vein, lymphatics and nerves enter or leave the apex of the pyramid at the hilum of the lung. Within each pulmonary segment the bronchus divides into numerous branches which follow one of two pathways; either an axial pathway which runs from the hilum of the lung to the pleural surface or a lateral pathway supplying the lung on either side of the axial pathways. The bronchi become progressively narrower and eventually become *bronchioles* which do not contain cartilage or mucous glands in their walls. The bronchioles divide further until the *terminal bronchioles* are reached; these lead into *respiratory bronchioles* which have *alveolar ducts* and *alveoli* opening into their lumen. Each respiratory bronchiole supplies about 200 alveoli.

Acinus

An acinus is the lung tissue distal to a terminal bronchiole and is composed of respiratory bronchioles and the alveolar ducts and alveoli which arise from them. It is a functioning unit of lung tissue. A *secondary lobule* comprises three to five acini.

Alveoli

There are 300 million alveoli in each lung and the average diameter of an alveolus at full inflation is 250 μ. The alveolar wall is 5 to 10 μ at the thinnest point and is composed of a continuous layer of epithelial cells, fibres of elastin, reticulin and collagen, and small arteries and capillaries.

Electron microscopy has shown that the epithelial lining of the alveoli consists of a continuous basement membrane and two types of cells called pneumocytes. Type 1 pneumocytes are predominant and are in direct contact with the pulmonary capillaries and contribute to the blood-gas barrier. The precise mechanism of gas diffusion across these cells is not known. Type II pneumocytes are responsible for the production of pulmonary surfactant. Small arteries and a meshwork of capillaries composed of endothelial cells lying on a continuous basement membrane form the other half of the blood-gas barrier.

Pores in the alveolar wall, pores of Kohn, allow collateral ventilation of air from alveolus to alveolus and segment to segment and help to prevent lobular and segmental collapse.

Pulmonary surfactant

Pulmonary surfactant is a surface tension lowering agent which lines the alveoli and is a liquid containing phospholipids. Surfactant reduces the surface tension of the alveolar walls and decreases the work required to expand the lungs. Without surfactant the alveoli would tend to collapse. Absence or inactivation of surfactant is probably responsible for the respiratory distress syndrome (hyaline membrane disease) in neonates. The respiratory distress syndrome may rarely occur in adults following severe trauma, shock or fat embolism. Prolonged inhalation of >40 per cent oxygen, cigarette smoke or noxious gases may inactivate surfactant.

Intra-alveolar macrophages

Macrophages are found within the alveoli. They come from the liver and spleen, and their function is to ingest bacteria and particulate matter which enter the alveoli.

Pulmonary circulation

The lung has a double blood supply from the pulmonary and bronchial arteries. The main pulmonary artery arises from the right ventricle and divides into right and left pulmonary arteries which branch in parallel with the bronchial tree and carry venous blood to the capillary bed adjacent to the alveoli of each lung. Here gas exchange takes place and the oxygenated blood returns through the pulmonary veins to the left atrium. The bronchial arteries arise from the thoracic aorta or from its intrathoracic branches and deliver arterial blood to the bronchial tree. At the level of the respiratory bronchioles the capillary beds of the bronchial and pulmonary arteries are continuous with each other and drain into the pulmonary veins. The bronchial veins receive venous blood from the larger bronchi in the hilar region and return it to the right atrium via the azygos vein.

The pulmonary and bronchial arteries accompany the bronchus in a common bronco-arterial bundle which runs centrally through each pulmonary segment. The pulmonary veins lie at the periphery each segment and mark its lateral boundaries. They mark the line of cleavage used to carry out a segmental resection.

The walls of the main pulmonary arteries and their larger branches contain muscle and elastic laminae. Arterioles contain little or no muscle and consist of collagen and a few elastic fibres.

Lymphatics

The lung has an abundant lymphatic supply which acts as a defence barrier against inhaled bacteria and particulate matter. There are numerous lymphatics around the bronchi, arteries, veins and pleura. The direction of lymphatic flow is from the periphery of the lung towards the hilum. Lymph nodes are situated between the bronchial bifurcations, in the main carina and along the trachea. Lymphatics from the right lung drain into the right paratracheal nodes. These nodes also receive lymph from the lower part of the left lower lobe via the subcarinal nodes. Lymphatics from the left upper lobe drain into the left paratracheal nodes. The lingula and the apical segment of the left lower lobe drain into both right and left paratracheal nodes. Lymph from the right paratracheal nodes enters the right lymphatic duct while on the left side lymph drains into the thoracic duct. Both vessels empty into the innominate veins.

Innervation

The trachea, bronchi and lungs are supplied by the vagus and the thoracic sympathetic nerves. Stimulation of the vagus causes broncho-constriction while sympathetic stimulation with drugs such as isoprenaline and adrenaline causes bronchial dilatation.

Pleura

The pleura is a thin connective tissue membrane lined by squamous epithelium. There are two layers of pleura; the visceral pleura, which lines the surface of the lung, and the parietal pleura, which lines the chest wall, mediastinum and the diaphragm. At the hilum the visceral pleura is continuous with the parietal pleura. The visceral and parietal pleura are separated by a thin film of fluid. This fluid arises from the subpleural capillaries and is absorbed by the pleural lymphatics. The space between the layers of pleura is known as the pleural space, but it becomes evident only if excessive fluid accumulates in the space (pleural effusion) or if air enters the space (pneumothorax). The pressure in the pleural space is subatmospheric and is produced by the elastic recoil of the lungs towards the hilum.

The visceral pleura is not sensitive to painful stimuli. Irritation of the parietal pleura causes pleuritic pain, which is felt at the site of involvement except when the pleura overlying the central part of the diaphragm is affected. This is supplied by the phrenic nerve which arises from the 3rd, 4th and 5th cervical nerves and the pain is referred to the shoulder tip.

Defence mechanisms of the respiratory tract

The integrity of the lungs is maintained by the defence mechanisms which have been mentioned previously. These include the gag and cough reflexes, the mucus secreting ciliated columnar epithelium, the lymphatics of the lung and the intra-alveolar macrophages.

In addition the lungs are protected by specific immunological defence mechanisms. The chief protective antibody of the bronchial secretions is IgA which is produced by plasma cells in the respiratory tract. IgA in bronchial secretions and saliva has an additional peptide chain, the secretory piece, which distinguishes it from IgA in the circulation. The secretory piece has a protective function and IgA in bronchial secretions is active in complement fixing antigen-antibody reactions. IgG and IgM also play a vital role in protection against common bacterial infections. Antibody deficiency states predispose to recurrent infections with common bacteria, eg. *Streptococcus pneumoniae* and *Staphylococcus aureus*.

Specific lymphocyte sensitization is also important, especially in immunity from tuberculosis. Deficiencies of cell mediated immunity predispose to severe infections with viruses and fungi. It is emphasized that antibody deficiency states and disorders of cell mediated immunity are uncommon.

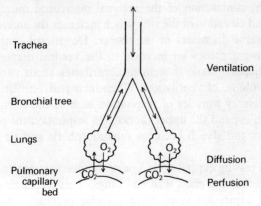

Fig. 2 Pulmonary function.

PULMONARY FUNCTION

The primary function of the lung is to add oxygen to the arterial blood and to remove carbon dioxide. This involves three fundamental processes (Fig. 2):

1. *Ventilation*: The movement of air in and out of the lungs.

2. *Perfusion*: The blood flow through the pulmonary capillary bed.

3. *Diffusion*: The transfer of oxygen and carbon dioxide between the terminal airways and alveoli and the pulmonary capillary blood.

The *volume* and *distribution* of ventilation and perfusion within the lungs is of major importance. Ventilation must supply an adequate volume of air and this must be distributed evenly to the perfused alveoli. Likewise, perfusion must be adequate in volume and must be distributed evenly to the ventilated alveoli. If these conditions are fulfilled, efficient gas exchange takes place and the partial pressures of oxygen (P_aO_2) and carbon dioxide (P_aCO_2) in the arterial blood are maintained within normal limits. The P_aO_2 is influenced by age and in young people the normal range is 85 to 100 mmHg while in healthy people over the age of 60 the normal range is 75 to 90 mmHg. The normal range for P_aCO_2 is 36 to 44 mmHg.

Ventilation

Ventilation consists of two phases, inspiration and expiration. On inspiration, contraction of the external intercostal muscles causes rotation and elevation of the ribs which increases the anteroposterior and transverse diameters of the thorax. Downward contraction of the diaphragm causes an increase in the vertical diameter of the thorax. Diaphragmatic movement contributes about two thirds of the total volume of ventilation. When increased ventilation is necessary accessory muscles of respiration such as the sternomastoids and scaleni expand the upper thorax. On inspiration the pressure in the airways and alveoli becomes subatmospheric and air flows into the lungs.

Normal resting expiration is a passive movement produced by the elastic recoil of the chest wall and lungs. This forces air out of the lungs and expiration stops when alveolar pressure equals atmospheric pressure. The abdominal wall muscles are used to achieve forced expiration.

Control of ventilation

The rhythm, rate and depth of breathing is controlled by the respiratory centre in the reticular formation of the medulla. Inspiration and expiration are regulated by different parts of the respiratory centre. Ventilation is modified by afferent impulses from neural receptors in the lungs and chest wall, and chemoreceptors in the medulla and in the carotid and aortic bodies.

Ventilation is regulated chiefly by the P_aCO_2. A rise in P_aCO_2 produces a fall in pH of the arterial blood and cerebrospinal fluid which stimulates the chemoreceptors in the medulla causing increased ventilation. The respiratory centre is not stimulated directly by changes in P_aO_2. The chemoreceptors in the aortic and carotid bodies are sensitive to changes in P_aO_2, P_aCO_2 and pH. A fall in P_aO_2 and to a lesser extent a rise in P_aCO_2 or fall in pH increase ventilation by stimulating the aortic and carotid chemoreceptors which are connected with the respiratory centre by the glossopharyngeal and vagus nerves.

In patients with severe chronic bronchitis the medullary chemoreceptors may become accustomed to raised p_aCO_2 levels and in these patients the main stimulus to ventilation is hypoxaemia. The hypoxic drive to respiration is removed by giving high concentrations of oxygen and this may result in further hypoventilation and increased retention of carbon dioxide.

Lung volumes and capacities
These are anatomical measurements which are affected by exercise and disease (Fig. 3).

Lung volumes. There are four primary lung volumes:

1. *Tidal volume* (TV) is the colume of air breathed in or out of the respiratory tract with each breath.
2. *Inspiratory reserve colume* (IRV) is the maximum volume of air which can be inspired from the resting inspiratory level.

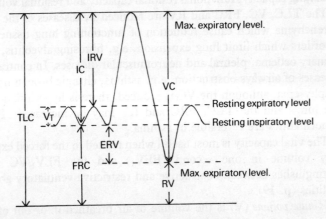

Fig. 3 Spirogram tracing showing lung volumes and capacities.

3. *Expiratory reserve volume* (ERV) is the maximum volume of air which can be expired from the resting expiratory level.
4. *Residual volume* (RV) is the volume of air remaining in the lungs at the end of a maximum expiration.

Lung capacities. There are four lung capacities, each of which includes two or more of the primary volumes.

1. *Total lung capacity* (TLC) is the volume of air contained in the lungs at the end of a maximum inspiration.
2. *Vital capacity* (VC) is the maximum volume of air that can be expired after a maximum inspiration.
3. *Inspiratory capacity* (IC) is the maximum volume of air that can be inspired from the resting expiratory level.
4. *Functional residual capacity* (FRC) is the volume of air remaining in the lungs at the resting expiratory level.

The tidal volume, inspiratory reserve volume, expiratory reserve volume, vital capacity and inspiratory capacity can be measured directly with a spirometer. The functional residual capacity is measured by indirect means using helium or nitrogen, and the residual volume and total lung capacity are then derived arithmetically. Individual values for lung volumes and capacities depend upon age, sex and height. Results are compared with predicted normal values; results may vary by as much as 20 per cent from the predicted values, although in a single individual repeated measurements differ by only 5 per cent.

In practice the most useful lung volumes are the vital capacity, total lung capacity, functional residual capacity and residual volume.

The TLC, VC, FRC and RV are reduced by diseases of the lung parenchyma which cause reduction of functioning lung tissue and disorders which limit lung expansion, e.g. fibrosing alveolitis, pulmonary oedema, pleural and neuromuscular diseases. In contrast in diseases of airways obstruction, e.g. asthma, chronic bronchitis and emphysema, although the VC is reduced, there is hyperinflation of the lungs and the TLC, FRC and RV may be increased. These abnormalities are reversible in asthma.

The vital capacity is most useful when related to the forced expiratory volume in one second (FEV_1) and the FEV_1/VC ratio distinguishes between obstructive and restrictive ventilatory abnormalities (p. 19).

Minute volume ($\dot{V}$) is the volume of air breathed in or out of the respiratory tract each minute. At rest the minute volume is about 6 l/min but it may increase to 70 l/min during heavy exercise. The minute volume can be measured by collecting expired air and dividing the volume collected by the number of minutes taken to collect the sample.

Respiratory frequency (f) or respiratory rate is the number of breaths taken per minute. At rest the respiratory rate is about 12, increasing to over 30 on exercise.

Tidal volume is about 500 ml at rest but may increase to 3 l during heavy exercise. The tidal volume is obtained by dividing the minute volume by the respiratory rate.

Anatomical dead space is the internal volume of the conducting airways from the nose and mouth to the alveoli and is about 150 ml.

Physiological dead space (VD) is the volume of inspired air which does not take part in gas exchange and it may be regarded as wasted ventilation. This includes the air contained in the conducting airways and in health the physiological dead space is only slightly greater than the anatomical dead space. The ratio between dead space ventilation and tidal volume (VD/VT)does not normally exceed 30 per cent in healthy young men at rest but may increase to 40 per cent in older subjects. The physiological dead space increases if ventilated alveoli are underperfused e.g. pulmonary embolism.

Alveolar ventilation ($\dot{V}$A) is the volume of fresh air entering the alveoli per minute. Alveolar ventilation is a better index of ventilation than minute volume or tidal volume, since it takes into account the volume of air wasted in ventilating the physiological dead space. At rest alveolar ventilation is about 4.5 l/min.

The $P_a CO_2$ is the best index of the efficiency of alveolar ventilation and it remains normal only if alveolar ventilation is adequate. The $P_a O_2$ is a less reliable index because it is adversely affected by ventilation-perfusion imbalance.

Hypoventilation: ventilatory failure
Hypoventilation is present when alveolar ventilation is insufficient to meet the metabolic requirements of the body. The term hypoventilation is synonymous with ventilatory failure (p. 143). Hypoventilation causes a rise in $P_a CO_2$ (hypercapnia) and a fall in $P_a O_2$ (hypoxaemia). The $P_a O_2$ falls because the partial pressure of oxygen in the alveoli is reduced. The rise in $P_a CO_2$ causes a fall in the pH of the blood which is called *respiratory acidosis*. Figure 21 shows the causes of ventilatory failure.

Hyperventilation
Hyperventilation is present when ventilation is greater than that normally required to keep the $P_a O_2$ and $P_a CO_2$ normal. Hyperven-

tilation reduces the alveolar PCO_2 and increased amounts of carbon dioxide pass from the pulmonary capillary blood to the alveoli, producing a fall in P_aCO_2 and a rise in pH which is termed *respiratory alkalosis*. In time the kidney compensates for the alkalosis by increased excretion of bicarbonate.

Hyperventilation increases the alveolar PO_2, and the P_aO_2 and arterial oxygen saturation rise if they are initially low. If the arterial oxygen saturation is normal, hyperventilation has little effect because of the sigmoid shape of the oxygen dissociation curve. Blood leaving normally ventilated alveoli is almost fully saturated with oxygen and any increase in the alveolar PO_2 produced by hyperventilation will not significantly increase the arterial oxygen saturation.

Hyperventilation occurs in response to stimulation of the respiratory centre and the aortic and carotid body chemoreceptors, and as a result of stimulation of stretch receptors and vascular baroreceptors in the lung. Hyperventilation is common in asthma, pneumonia, fibrosing alveolitis, pulmonary embolism and metabolic acidosis. Hyperventilation is occasionally due to neurosis.

Perfusion
At rest the cardiac output is 5 l/min and this volume of blood passes through the pulmonary capillary bed to be oxygenated. In the erect position, due to the effect of gravity, perfusion ($\dot{Q}$) increases in linear fashion from the top to the bottom of the lung and is greatest in the lower zones. Alveolar perfusion is reduced in pulmonary embolism and in diseases which cause obliteration of the pulmonary capillary bed such as chronic bronchitis and fibrosing alveolitis. These disorders may cause pulmonary hypertension if more than two thirds of the pulmonary vascular bed is obliterated.

Distribution of ventilation and perfusion
In normal persons at rest with alveolar ventilation 4.5 l/min and perfusion 5 l/min, the average ventilation-perfusion ratio ($\dot{V}_A/\dot{Q}$) of the lung as a whole is 0.9. However, some alveoli are ventilated but not perfused and have a ventilation-perfusion ratio of infinity while others are perfused but not ventilated and have a ventilation-perfusion ratio of zero. Between these two extremes there is a great variety of ventilation-perfusion ratios. For the purposes of understanding ventilation-perfusion imbalance it is convenient to consider the lung as if it were divided into three compartments.

1. A compartment in which the alveoli are normally ventilated and perfused and $\dot{V}_A/\dot{Q} = 0.9$.

2. A compartment in which alveoli are well ventilated but poorly perfused and $\dot{V}A/\dot{Q}$ is high. Because of the wasted ventilation this compartment acts as *physiological dead space (dead space effect)*. Blood leaving regions of the lung with high ventilation-perfusion ratios has a supernormal P_aO_2 and low P_aCO_2. Diseases which cause local reduction of perfusion and high ventilation-perfusion ratios include pulmonary embolism and fibrosing alveolitis. High ventilation-perfusion ratios never occur as an isolated abnormality because blood is diverted to other regions of the lung, where increased perfusion relative to ventilation results in hypoxaemia which is the characteristic effect of these diseases.

3. A compartment in which alveoli are poorly ventilated but well perfused and $\dot{V}A/\dot{Q}$ is low. This compartment acts as a *physiological shunt* because mixed venous blood bypasses the alveoli (*venous admixture effect*).

Blood leaving alveoli which are poorly ventilated has a low P_aO_2 and raised P_aCO_2. A rise in P_aCO_2 of the mixed arterial blood will cause compensatory hyperventilation in other regions of lung and this maintains the overall P_aCO_2 within normal limits or may even produce a fall in P_aCO_2. Hyperventilation will not compensate for hypoxaemia because blood leaving normally ventilated alveoli is almost fully saturated with oxygen Reduction in ventilation-perfusion ratio is the single most important cause of hypoxaemia but can be corrected by the administration of oxygen. Diseases which cause reduction in ventilation-perfusion ratios include pneumonia, pulmonary collapse, pulmonary oedema, fibrosing alveolitis, asthma and chronic bronchitis and emphysema.

Diffusion

Diffusion is the process whereby oxygen and carbon dioxide are transferred across the alveolar capillary membrane. Diffusion depends on the difference between the partial pressures of the gas on either side of the membrane. The rate of gas transfer for a pressure difference of 1 mmHg is called the *diffusing capacity* (DL) or *transfer factor* (TL).

Carbon monoxide is used routinely for measurement of diffusing capacity (DLCO) because of its great affinity for haemoglobin which means that little remains dissolved in the blood plasma to exert any back pressure.

Carbon monoxide uptake is measured either during tidal breathing ('steady state' method) or while holding breath for 10 seconds at full lung inflation ('single breath' method). The patient inhales gas containing a low concentration of carbon monoxide, and the concentration of carbon monoxide in the mixed expired gas is measured. The difference between these two concentrations is a measure of the amount of carbon monoxide which has been transferred across the alveolar capillary membrane. The normal values for diffusing capacity depend on age, sex, height and the method used for its assessment. Using the single breath method the diffusing capacity is about 25 ml/min/mmHg.

The diffusing capacity is low in emphysema because of reduction in the effective alveolar surface area available for gas exchange. It is also reduced in parenchymal diseases which involve the interstitial tissues such as sarcoidosis, fibrosing alveolitis and allergic alveolitis. In these diseases reduction in total lung capacity and ventilation-perfusion imbalance are the main factors responsible for defective gas transfer, increased thickness of the alveolar capillary membrane being a relatively minor factor.

Oxygen transport

Transport of gases is related to pressure gradients; gases move from a point of high concentration or high pressure to one of low concentration or low pressure. The partial pressure of oxygen falls progressively from a level of 150 mmHg in air, to 100 mmHg in alveolar gas, 98 mmHg in arterial blood and 40 mmHg in mixed venous blood. This pressure gradient drives oxygen from the alveoli into the pulmonary capillary blood. In the tissues the arterial blood gives up oxygen because of the lower tissue partial pressure of oxygen. Important factors which influence oxygen delivery to the tissues are the arterial oxygen concentration and the total and regional blood flow.

Oxygen is transported from the lungs to the tissues chemically combined with haemoglobin and a small amount is carried in solution. The oxyhaemoglobin dissociation curve (Fig. 4) is sigmoid shaped and in the upper range, despite a moderate fall in partial pressure of oxygen, the arterial oxygen saturation remains high. Thus a fall in partial pressure from 100 to 60 mmHg produces only a 6 per cent drop in oxygen saturation from 96 to 90 per cent. This means that despite low oxygen tensions the haemoglobin delivered to the tissues remains almost fully saturated with oxygen. When the partial pressure falls below 60 mmHg there is a marked fall in arterial oxygen saturation and further small reductions in tension produce large falls in saturation. Reduction in pH, carbon dioxide retention and increase in temperature shift the curve to the right and help to release oxygen from haemoglobin to meet the metabolic demands of the tissues.

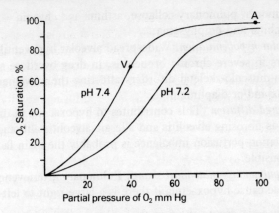

Fig. 4 Oxyhaemoglobin dissociation curve relating the partial pressure of oxygen to the percentage oxygen saturation, blood pH 7.4 and temperature 37°C. Acidosis, hypercapnia and fever shift the curve to the right. V = mixed venous blood; A = arterial blood.

It can be seen that transport of oxygen is affected by many factors including the partial pressure of inspired oxygen, alveolar ventilation, diffusion across the alveolar capillary membrane, distribution of ventilation and perfusion, cardiac output, haemoglobin content, acid-base disorders and temperature.

Hypoxaemia.

Hypoxaemia is present when the partial pressure of oxygen in the arterial blood is less than normal (p. 145). P_aO_2 levels decrease with age and are affected by the care with which the sample of blood is obtained. Arterial blood is usually obtained by radial or brachial artery puncture after adequate local anaesthesia. Blood is collected in a heparinized syringe. Any air which enters the syringe must be expelled and the end of the syringe is then sealed from the atmosphere. The syringe is rotated to mix the sample and if analysis cannot be done immediately the syringe should be placed on a tray of ice. The site of the arterial puncture should be compressed for at least three minutes after withdrawing the needle.

In patients with respiratory disease the P_aO_2 is one indication of the degree of functional abnormality. In severe respiratory failure the P_aO_2 may fall to 30–40 mmHg.

Hypoxaemia due to respiratory disease is caused by one or more of the following mechanisms.

1. *Ventilation-perfusion imbalance.* The commonest cause of hypoxaemia is reduction in ventilation-perfusion ratio, e.g.

pneumonia, pulmonary collapse, asthma and chronic bronchitis and emphysema.

2. *Alveolar hypoventilation*. Widespread alveolar hypoventilation occurs in severe chronic bronchitis, in drug overdose and in neuro-musculo-skeletal disorders affecting the movement of the thorax and/or diaphragm.

3. *Impaired diffusion*. This contributes to hypoxaemia in diseases such as fibrosing alveolitis and allergic alveolitis although ventilation-perfusion imbalance is probably the main factor responsible.

4. *Intrapulmonary anatomical shunts*. Pulmonary arteriovenous fistulae cause hypoxaemia if there is a large right to left shunt.

Hypoxaemia due to the first three abnormalities is corrected by breathing 100 per cent oxygen. In practice 30 per cent oxygen is usually sufficient to raise the P_aO_2 to normal levels. Hypoxaemia due to a large right to left intrapulmonary shunt is not corrected by breathing 100 per cent oxygen.

Hypoxaemia may also be caused by:

Cardiac disease, e.g. right to left intracardiac shunt due to congenital heart disease.

Deficiency of oxygen in inspired air, e.g. altitude, caves.

Carbon dioxide transport

Carbon dioxide produced by tissue metabolism is excreted by the lungs. The partial pressure of carbon dioxide in the tissues is greater than the partial pressure in the arterial blood. This creates a gradient so that carbon dioxide diffuses from the tissues into the blood. Carbon dioxide is transported in the blood in three forms: as dissolved carbon dioxide, as carbamino compounds and as bicarbonate. Some carbon dioxide forms carbamino compounds in the plasma with the amino group of plasma proteins but a larger proportion forms carbamino compounds in the red cell with the amino group of haemoglobin. Carbon dioxide is also transported as bicarbonate in the plasma and the enzyme carbonic anhydrase contained in the red cell catalyses the following:

$$CO_2 + H_2O \rightleftarrows H_2CO_3 \rightleftarrows H^+ + HCO_3'$$

The hydrogen ions are buffered by the reduced haemoglobin in capillary blood because reduced haemoglobin is a better buffer than oxyhaemoglobin. The reaction is facilitated by the simultaneous dissociation of oxyhaemoglobin and the transfer of oxygen from capillary blood to the tissues. Bicarbonate accumulates within the red cell and most diffuses into the plasma and is replaced by chloride cations from the plasma in order to maintain electrical neutrality of the red cell (chloride shift).

In the pulmonary capillaries the reverse reaction takes place and oxygen is taken up and carbon dioxide is unloaded. Conversion of reduced haemoglobin to oxyhaemoglobin releases hydrogen ions which combine with bicarbonate ions to form carbonic acid which then breaks down into carbon dioxide and water. Carbon dioxide leaves the red cells and passes from the mixed venous blood where its partial pressure is 46 mmHg to the alveoli where the partial pressure is 40 mmHg.

The amount of carbon dioxide carried by the blood is related to its partial pressure, and the relationship between carbon dioxide content and partial pressure is almost linear in the physiological range.

Hypercapnia
Hypercapnia is present when the partial pressure of carbon dioxide in the arterial blood is above the upper limit of normal ie 44 mmHg. The cause of hypercapnia is alveolar hypoventilation (p. 143). Severe alveolar hypoventilation is present if the P_aCO_2 exceeds 70 mmHg. The effects of hypercapnia are discussed on page 145.

Acid-base balance
The lung plays an important role in the regulation of the blood pH by excreting carbon dioxide. The kidneys are mainly responsible for regulating the concentration of bicarbonate ions, but respond more slowly to changes in pH than the lungs. Figure 22 summarizes the relationship between pH, bicarbonate and P_aCO_2. Retention of carbon dioxide causes respiratory acidosis while excessive excretion of carbon dioxide results in respiratory alkalosis.

Mechanics of breathing
Breathing involves the expenditure of energy to overcome the inertia of the lungs and chest wall, their elastic and viscous resistance to movement and the frictional resistance to air flow through the trachea and bronchi. The work of breathing increases if there is increased stiffness of the lungs or increased airway resistance and these are the main factors responsible for dyspnoea.

Compliance
The compliance of the lung is a measure of the distensibility of the lung and is defined as the volume change per unit pressure change.

It is determined by measuring the intrapleural pressure change, recorded with an oesophageal ballon, and the volume change produced by different levels of lung inflation. Measurements are made either during normal breathing (dynamic compliance) or during breath-holding (static compliance). The normal range for pulmonary compliance is 0.08–0.33 l per cm H_2O. A lung with low compliance expands less than one with high compliance when both are inflated by the same pressure.

Lung compliance is reduced by diseases which increase the stiffness of the lung and limit expansion, e.g. pulmonary oedema, pulmonary collapse, pneumonia, fibrosing alveolitis, lymphangitis carcinomatosa and pleural effusion. Chest wall compliance is reduced in kyphoscoliosis and ankylosing spondylitis.

Airway resistance

The airway resistance is the frictional resistance to air flow through the airways and can be measured using a body plethysmograph. Airway resistance is increased in asthma, chronic bronchitis and emphysema. In routine practice, measurement of FEV_1/FVC or PEFR are used to detect the presence of increased resistance or obstruction to airflow (PEFR: peak expiratory flow rate, p. 20).

Ventilatory capacity

Forced expiratory volume (FEV) is the volume of air breathed out in standard time during a maximum forced expiration following a maximum inspiration. Usually the FEV is measured during the first second of a forced expiration; this is termed the FEV_1. The FEV_1 is a most useful index of the severity of impairment of ventilatory capacity. An FEV_1 of <1 l indicates severe impairment of function.

Forced vital capacity (FVC) is the total volume of air breathed out during a maximum forced expiration following a maximum inspiration. Normally the FVC is nearly the same as the VC but it may be less in patients with airways obstruction because of premature closure of the airways with consequent air trapping. The FVC is reduced in a large number of conditions (p. 21) and it is useful index of the severity of functional impairment in diffuse parenchymal disease of the lungs.

The FEV_1 and FVC are measured with a spirometer and portable instruments such as the Vitalograph are easy to use and give rapid and reliable results. It is essential that the technique is explained carefully to the patient and he should be encouraged to blow as hard and as fast as possible after a maximum inspiration. It is usual to record the best value of two or three attempts. Predicted normal values depend upon the patient's age, sex and height.

The FEV_1 should always be related to the FVC or VC. Healthy young people can expel about 80 per cent of the FVC in 1 second and the FEV_1/FVC ratio is about 80 per cent (Fig. 5). In normal people over 70 years of age the ratio may be as low as 60 per cent. The FEV_1/FVC ratio is of great value in differentiating between diseases which cause airways obstruction and diseases which diffusely involve the lung parenchyma.

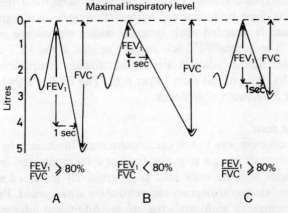

Maximal inspiratory level

Fig. 5 (A) Normal spirogram; (B) Spirogram showing obstructive ventilatory defect with marked reduction in FEV_1 and FEV_1/FVC ratio less than 80%. (C) Spirogram showing restrictive ventilatory defect with proportionate reduction in both FEV_1 and FVC so that the FEV_1/FVC ratio is greater than 80%.

Obstructive ventilatory defect
Diseases which cause airways obstruction, such as asthma, chronic bronchitis and emphysema, cause a greater reduction in FEV_1 than FVC so that the FEV_1/FVC ratio is less than 80 per cent (Fig. 5); sometimes the ratio falls to 30 per cent or less. Ventilatory capacity may improve after treatment with bronchodilators and corticosteroids, and assessment of reversibility of airways obstruction is used for the selection of appropriate therapy in these diseases (p. 120).

Restrictive ventilatory defect
In diseases of the lung parenchyma such as sarcoidosis, fibrosing alveolitis and allergic alveolitis the FEV_1 and FVC are both reduced in the same proportion and the FEV_1/FVC ratio remains about 80 per cent (Fig. 5). This is called a restrictive ventilatory defect. This type of defect also occurs when lung expansion is reduced by pul-

monary collapse, pneumonia, pleural effusion or chest wall abnormalities such as ankylosing spondylitis.

Peak expiratory flow rate (PEFR) is the maximum flow rate during a maximum expiration and may be easily measured with a portable Wright peak flow meter. Normal values for young men are about 600 l/min and for women 400 l/min. Airways obstruction causes reduction in PEFR and in severe cases it is less than 100 l/min. PEFR is useful in assessing severity and monitoring progress of airways obstruction.

Forced expiratory time (FET) is the time taken for a person to empty the chest by forced expiration following a maximum inspiration, and is recorded while listening with a stethoscope over the trachea. The normal FET is 4 seconds or less. If the FET is more than 6 seconds it indicates airways obstruction comparable to an FEV_1/FVC ratio of less than 50 per cent. The FET is a useful bedside test for airways obstruction.

Exercise tests
A most effective way to test cardiopulmonary function is by means of exercise tests using a step, treadmill or cycle ergometer. In a simple exercise test the work load is progressively increased and the heart rate, electrocardiogram and ventilation are recorded. Performance is compared with predicted values. Additional information is obtained by analysis of expired air and arterial blood obtained during exercise.

SUMMARY

A basic knowledge of respiratory physiology is helpful in understanding the clinical features of certain diseases and the role of pulmonary function tests in diagnosis and management.

Pulmonary function tests are used to assess the severity and type of functional impairment, the effects of treatment and the course of the disease. The characteristic patterns of altered function which occur in diseases causing airways obstruction and diseases of the lung parenchyma are shown in Table 1.

The most useful tests of pulmonary function and the main indications for their use are summarized as follows:
1. *FEV_1 and FVC.* Measurement of FEV_1 and FVC is used to determine ventilatory capacity and to distinguish between diseases causing obstructive and restrictive ventilatory defects (p. 19). Ventilatory capacity is measured preoperatively in patients with respiratory disability especially before thoracic surgery (p. 174). FEV_1 and FVC are also used to assess

Table 1 Characteristic patterns of pulmonary function in diseases causing airways obstruction and diseases of the lung parenchyma.

	Airways obstruction: Asthma, chronic bronchitis, emphysema	Parenchymal diseases: Sarcoidosis, fibrosing alveolitis, allergic alveolitis
Ventilatory capacity		
FEV_1	↓	N or ↓
FVC	N or ↓	↓
FEV_1/FVC	↓ (<80%) obstructive	N (>80%) restrictive
Lung volumes		
TLC	N or ↑	↓
FRC	↑	↓
RV	↑	↓
Transfer factor		
TLCO	Asthma N	↓
	Chron. bron. N	
	Emphysema ↓	
Blood gas analysis		
PaO_2	↓	↓
$PaCo_2$	Asthma N or ↓	N or ↓
	Chron. bron. N or ↑	
	Emphysema N or ↓	

N = normal;   ↓ = decreased or tends to decrease;   ↑ = increased or tends to increase

progress and the efficacy of bronchodilator and corticosteroid therapy (p. 120). All students should be able to measure FEV_1 and FVC.

2. *Lung volumes.* These measurements are mainly used in the assessment of diseases of the lung parenchyma such as sarcoidosis and fibrosing alveolitis.

3. *Transfer factor.* This is a useful measurement of functional impairment in parenchymal diseases.

4. *Blood gas analysis.* Estimations of P_aO_2, P_aCO_2 and pH are used to determine the efficiency of pulmonary function and are essential in the management of patients with respiratory failure (p. 145) or severe asthma.

FURTHER READING

Bates D V, Macklem P T, Christie R V 1971 Respiratory function in disease. 2nd edn. Saunders Philadelphia

Comroe J H, Forster R E, Dubois A B, Briscoe W A, Carlsen E 1962 The lung clinical physiology and pulmonary function tests. 2nd edn. Year Book Chicago.

Cotes J E 1979 Lung function. 4th edn. Blackwell, Oxford

Freedman S 1981 Lung function tests. Hospital Update, March, 281

West J B 1979 Respiratory physiology: The essentials. 2nd edn. Blackwell, Oxford

2

Classification of respiratory diseases

Respiratory diseases may be classified on an aetiological, anatomical or pathophysiological basis. None of these classifications is entirely satisfactory because the aetiological agents are unknown in some diseases while in others the same causal agent may affect different anatomical sites and produce different pathophysiological effects. A classification based solely on changes in structure and function also has practical disadvantages. The following broad classification serves only as an introduction to subsequent chapters and in practice it is preferable to think in terms of specific diseases.

Infections of the respiratory tract
Respiratory infections are mainly caused by bacteria, viruses, or *Mycoplasma pneumoniae*. Rickettsial and fungal infections are relatively uncommon and are largely confined to certain geographical regions. Respiratory infections occur at any age but are commonest in the young, the elderly and the immunosuppressed. The clinical features are determined by the causal organism, the site of infection and whether the infection is acute or chronic.

Acute respiratory infections
Acute infections predominantly involve the upper respiratory tract, e.g. *coryza*, the bronchial tree, e.g. *acute bronchitis* or the lungs, e.g. *pneumonia, lung abscess.*

Chronic respiratory infections
Tuberculosis is the commonest chronic infection and mainly affects the lungs. *Bronchiectasis* is a chronic infection characterized by pathological dilatation of the bronchi. Chronic bronchitis also involves the bronchial tree and causes generalized narrowing of the airways. However, infection is not the main aetiological factor, nor are the clinical signs of infection always present, and for these reasons it is best regarded as a disease of airways obstruction which emphasizes the cardinal abnormalities in structure and function.

Disease of airways obstruction

Bronchial asthma, chronic bronchitis and emphysema

Asthma and chronic bronchitis cause generalized narrowing of the airways due to excessive intrabronchial secretions, mucosal oedema and bronchial muscle spasm. Attacks of asthma are commonly precipitated by infection or inhalation of allergens. Asthma often begins in childhood, while chronic bronchitis, which is caused by cigarette smoking and atmospheric pollution, rarely develops before the age of 40.

Emphysema also causes airways obstruction and is characterized by increase beyond the normal in the size of the air spaces distal to the terminal bronchiole. It is usually associated with chronic bronchitis and arises after the age of 40.

Diseases of the pulmonary vessels

Pulmonary thromboembolism: pulmonary embolism and pulmonary infarction

Pulmonary embolism occurs when an embolus, usually a thrombus from the veins of the pelvis or lower limb, lodges in the pulmonary arterial tree. Pulmonary infarction is the term used to describe the pathological changes which may develop in the lung after an artery is obstructed by an embolus or by local thrombosis. These related disorders are collectively termed pulmonary thromboembolism. Many factors predispose to thromboembolism and it occurs most commonly over the age of 40.

Neoplastic diseases

Bronchial carcinoma

Bronchial carcinoma is the commonest neoplasm of the respiratory tract and is strongly associated with cigarette smoking. The lungs and pleura are sometimes the site of metastatic malignancy.

Occupational lung diseases

These diseases are the result of occupational exposure to dusts, gases or fumes. Particles which measure 5μ or less in diameter may enter the alveoli and cause disease in the lung.

Pneumoconiosis

Continued inhalation of inorganic dust over many years may lead to the accumulation of dust in the lungs where it causes tissue reactions. The commonest types are coalworkers' pneumoconiosis, silicosis and asbestosis.

Extrinsic allergic alveolitis

Inhalation of certain organic dusts may cause a type III hypersensitivity reaction in the lung which is termed 'extrinic allergic alveolitis'. This is usually an acute disease and symptoms arise in a sensitized individual 4 to 6 hours after exposure to the casual allergen. Farmer's lung and Bird Fancier's lung are the commonest forms of allergic alveolitis.

Exposure to irritant gases or fumes may cause acute pulmonary oedema e.g. chlorine.

Occupational asthma

Asthma can occur as a result of exposure to industrial agents such as toluene di-isocyanate (TDI), platinum salts, epoxy resin hardener and red cedar sawdust.

Diseases of unknown aetiology

Sarcoidosis

Sarcoidosis is a systemic granulomatous disease which commonly affects the respiratory tract causing bilateral hilar lymphadenopathy and/or pulmonary lesions.

Fibrosing alveolitis

Fibrosing alveolitis is a form of diffuse pulmonary fibrosis which involves the interstitial tissues of the lung with characteristic histological, radiological and clinical features.

Collagen disorders

Occasionally the lungs and pleura are involved by collagen disorders such as rheumatoid arthritis, systemic lupus erythematosus, systemic sclerosis and polyarteritis nodosa.

Diseases of the pleura

Pleurisy

Inflammation of the pleura is termed pleurisy and is usually secondary to pneumonia or pulmonary infarction.

Pleural effusion

Pleural effusion is an accumulation of fluid in the pleural space and may be caused by many diseases. Pus in the pleural space is termed *empyema*.

Pneumothorax
This is the term given to a collection of air in the pleural space.

Mesothelioma
A malignant tumour of the pleura usually associated with previous exposure to blue asbestos.

3

History taking

RESPIRATORY SYMPTOMS

The main symptoms of respiratory disease are cough, sputum, hae-moptysis, breathlessness, wheeze and chest pain. Less common symptoms include hoarseness, stridor, postnasal drip and night sweats. Considered individually these symptoms are of little help in diagnosis but certain combinations of symptoms and their mode of onset have considerable diagnostic value. The physician must listen carefully to the patient's story and obtain a detailed account of each symptom. Table 2 is a guide for history taking.

Cough

Cough is the commonest respiratory symptom and is a protective reflex (p. 1). Cough may be caused by disease anywhere in the lower respiratory tract and may also be a symptom of upper respiratory tract disease. Cough may be dry or productive of sputum.

Cough of recent onset is usually due to upper respiratory tract infection, acute bronchitis or pneumonia.

Table 2 A guide for history taking

Respiratory symptoms	Past history
Cough	Tuberculosis, pneumonia, measles,
Sputum	pertussis
Haemoptysis	Previous treatment
Breathlessness	Penicillin allergy, corticosteroids
Wheeze	Family history
Chest pain	Tuberculosis, asthma
	Occupational history
Hoarseness	Farming, mining, industrial exposure
Stridor	Social history
Postnasal drip	Smoking, alcohol, pets, overseas travel
Night sweats	Previous chest radiographs

History taking always includes interrogation for symptoms caused by disease of other systems.

Persistent cough, particularly in middle age, may be due to chronic bronchitis, bronchial carcinoma, bronchiectasis, asthma or tuberculosis. The cough of chronic bronchitis is characteristically worse on walking and is accompanied by wheeze and expectoration of sputum. Bronchiectasis also causes productive cough which is troublesome on rising, but usually the cough dates from childhood and larger volumes of sputum are produced. Cough is common in tuberculosis when it may be accompanied by weight loss and night sweats. Persistent cough should never be ignored or merely attributed to cigarette smoking without excluding bronchial carcinoma or other serious disease by radiographic examination of the lungs.

Occasionally cough is a symptom of spontaneous pneumothorax. This should be suspected if the onset is sudden and there is breathlessness and pleuritic pain.

Cough is sometimes the first symptom in asthma and in mild attacks it may not be accompanied by wheeze. Patients with chronic postnasal drip commonly have a productive cough, but on questioning they will usually admit that the expectorations come from the back of the throat.

A fit of coughing may cause syncope. This is called cough syncope and it is probably due to transient cerebral hypoxaemia. Cough syncope occurs most commonly in chronic bronchitis. Occasionally the muscular effort of coughing fractures one of the lower ribs causing pain and tenderness which is localized to the affected rib.

Sputum

Sputum is the name given to expectorated bronchial secretions; sputum is not coughed up unless the bronchial secretions are excessive. Sputum may be mucoid, purulent, frothy, black or bloodstained.

Mucoid sputum occurs in asthma and in the early stages of chronic bronchitis but in both conditions the sputum may be purulent if infection is present.

Purulent sputum contains mucus, bacteria and varying numbers of pus cells. It is yellow or green in colour and is a sign of respiratory infection. Purulent sputum is common in pneumonia, chronic bronchitis, bronchiectasis and lung abscess. The sputum may be copious and foul-smelling in the latter two diseases. The 24-hour volume of sputum and the degree of purulence are used to assess the efficacy of antibiotic treatment in respiratory infections.

Frothy sputum which is mucoid and tinged with blood is characteristic of acute pulmonary oedema.

Black sputum is sometimes coughed up by coal miners and by city dwellers who live in areas with high atmospheric pollution. The black colour is due to carbon particles.

Haemoptysis

Haemoptysis is the term used to describe the coughing up of blood from the lower respiratory tract. Careful questioning may be necessary to differentiate haemoptysis from haematemesis. Haematemesis is the vomiting of blood and is usually preceded by nausea and the blood is mixed with vomitus. Haemoptysis is preceded by cough and the blood may be mixed with mucoid or purulent sputum which contains bubbles of air. The amount of blood coughed up varies from blood stained streaking of the sputum to a profuse life threatening haemorrhage.

Haemoptysis is common in bronchial carcinoma, tuberculosis and pulmonary infarction and is often the presenting symptom. Recurrent haemoptysis over many years is a feature of bronchiectasis. Slight haemoptysis may occur in pneumonia and during an exacerbation of chronic bronchitis. Haemoptysis is a serious symptom and a chest radiograph should always be taken. Bronchoscopy is often necessary when the cause of the haemoptysis is uncertain.

Breathlessness

Breathlessness is a common complaint and may be caused by respiratory disease, cardiac disease, anaemia or metabolic disorders such as diabetic ketoacidosis and renal failure. Breathlessness during exercise is normal, provided it is not disproportionate to the work load.

Breathlessness due to respiratory disease may be caused by disorders of the bronchi, lungs, pulmonary vessels or pleura:

Bronchi: Asthma, bronchitis.

Lungs: Pneumonia, pulmonary collapse, pulmonary fibrosis, emphysema.

Pulmonary vessels: Pulmonary thrombo-embolism.

Pleura: Pleural effusion, pneumothorax.

Dyspnoea is the term used to describe a subjective state in which there is awareness of breathing. The mechanism whereby a person becomes conscious of the effort of breathing is not clear.

It is important to ascertain the severity of the breathlessness and whether it is present at rest or only on exercise. The degree of exercise which causes breathlessness should be determined and it is convenient to record this as the number of steps the patient can climb or the distance he can walk or run before becoming breathless.

Breathlessness of sudden onset occurs in acute asthma, pulmonary oedema, pulmonary embolism, pneumothorax and after inhalation of a foreign body. In these conditions the breathlessness may begin within minutes. Acute asthma and acute pulmonary oedema cause paroxysmal attacks of breathlessness which commonly begin during the night. Pneumonia causes breathlessness which develops over a period of hours or days.

Breathlessness of gradual onset occurs in chronic bronchitis and emphysema, pneumoconiosis and fibrosing alveolitis. The breathlessness develops gradually over a number of years and only in retrospect may the patient realise that his exercise tolerance has diminished.

Wheeze

Wheeze is a whistling sound caused by air flowing through narrowed airways. It is a symptom of airways obstruction and occurs in asthma, chronic bronchitis and emphysema. The airways narrowing is caused by excessive secretions, mucosal oedema and bronchial muscle spasm. Wheeze is louder during expiration than inspiration because of the normal expiratory narrowing of the bronchial tree. Rhonchi are heard on auscultation in patients with wheeze. In asthma the wheeze often starts in childhood and is paroxysmal. Acute wheezing attacks commonly occur during the night and must be differentiated from paroxysmal nocturnal dyspnoea due to pulmonary oedema. The wheeze of chronic bronchitis and emphysema begins in middle age and is most troublesome on waking and on exertion, and its severity is fairly constant from week to week. Occasionally bronchial carcinoma or inhaled foreign body may partially occlude a bronchus and produce wheeze which is localized to a single lobe.

Chest pain

Pleuritic pain. This is the characteristic chest pain caused by respiratory disease. It is sharp in quality and is aggravated by coughing and deep breathing. Pleuritic pain is caused by irritation of the pleura and is usually due to pleurisy secondary to pneumonia or pulmonary infarction. Less common causes include spontaneous pneumothorax, malignant involvement of the pleura, rib fracture and pleurodynia. Irritation of the diaphragmatic pleura produces pain which is referred to the shoulder tip. Sometimes pleuritic pain is referred to the upper abdomen where it mimics peritoneal pain. A pleural rub is often heard on auscultation of the chest at the site of the pain.

Tracheal pain. Retrosternal soreness which is aggravated by coughing is a feature of tracheitis.

Mediastinal pain. Intrathoracic malignancy involving the mediastinum may cause pain which is aching in quality and is felt deep in the chest.

Chest wall pain. Rib fractures and neoplastic involvement of the ribs and intercostal nerves produce severe localized, superficial pain.

Chest pain may also be due to cardiac disease or may be referred to the chest from disease in the abdomen.

Hoarseness

Hoarseness is usually caused by laryngitis. Bronchial carcinoma or mediastinal tumours which involve the left recurrent laryngeal nerve may cause persistent hoarseness.

Stridor

Stridor is characterised by noisy inspiration and may be loud and croaking. It is due to obstruction of the larynx, trachea or main bronchi by inflammation, foreign body or tumour and always warrants urgent attention. The commonest cause is croup (laryngo-tracheo-bronchitis) in children. Diphtheria should be remembered as a cause of stridor although it is now uncommon in Western countries.

Postnasal drip

This is the term given to secretions which drip down the back of the pharynx from the upper air passages and it is usually a symptom of sinusitis or rhinitis. Postnasal drip is common in bronchiectasis because this disease is often accompanied by chronic sinusitis.

Night sweats

Night sweats are an important symptom since they may be a manifestation of tuberculosis. Tuberculosis should always be suspected if night sweats are persistent and profuse, especially if they cannot be attributed to the central heating or hot weather.

When a patient presents with certain respiratory symptoms it is important to enquire about other symptoms which signify respiratory disease and also symptoms caused by disease of other systems. In addition the patient is asked about his past medical history, previous treatment, family history, occupational history and social history.

Past medical history

It is important to enquire about a past history of pneumonia and tuberculosis. Recurrent pneumonia is sometimes a manifestation of bronchial carcinoma, bronchiectasis or immuno-logical disorders (p. 90). Tuberculosis is a chronic disease and may recur if the patient has not had antituberculosis chemotherapy or if treatment has been inadequate. Only if it can be established with certainty that previous chemotherapy satisfies certain criteria (p. 195) can it be assumed that the present illness is unlikely to be due to reactivation of tuberculosis. Measles and pertussis predispose to bronchiectasis and a previous history of these diseases is sometimes relevant in adults with persistent cough and purulent sputum. A history of recent surgery under general anaesthesia may be significant because pneumonia and pulmonary infarction are relatively common during the first or second postoperative weeks.

Previous treatment

Penicillins are commonly used in the treatment of respiratory infections and it is important to ascertain whether the patient is allergic to penicillin. Patients with wheeze are asked about previous treatment with corticosteroids and the effect this had upon the wheeze. The wheeze of asthma is usually relieved by corticosteroids, but these drugs have little effect in chronic bronchitis and emphysema. It is essential to obtain details of chemotherapy in patients previously treated for tuberculosis.

Family history

All patients should be asked whether members of their family, or other close contacts, have ever had tuberculosis. Because of its infectious nature, tuberculosis has a strong familial tendency. Even contact which occurred many years previously may be aetiologically important because tuberculosis in adults is usually due to reactivation of tuberculosis acquired in childhood.

A family history of asthma and allergy is more common in patients with asthma than in those with chronic bronchitis and this is one factor which may be helpful when deciding whether wheeze is due to asthma or chronic bronchitis and emphysema.

Occupational history

A detailed occupational history is particularly important in patients with diffuse radiographic abnormalities. Coalworkers' pneumoconiosis, silicosis and asbestosis are the commonest occupational diseases in this category and mainly occur in miners after prolonged exposure. Pleural mesothelioma is an occasional complication in asbestos miners and in workers who use blue asbestos in insulating processes. Mesothelioma develops more than 20 years after the initial exposure to blue asbestos and in many cases the degree of exposure is minimal.

Inhalation of organic dust causes allergic alveolitis of which the commonest type is farmer's lung. This presents as an acute illness in farmers working with mouldy hay. Inhalation of irritant gases used in industry may also cause acute respiratory disease. Certain chemicals e.g. TDI, colophony, may cause asthma.

Social history

It is very important to obtain details of the patient's smoking habits. The prevalence of bronchial carcinoma and chronic bronchitis and emphysema is high in smokers and extremely low in non-smokers. The individual risk of developing these diseases is directly related to the number of cigarettes smoked each day and the total number of years the habit is continued. Heavy alcohol intake predisposes to recurrent pneumonia. Budgerigars and pigeons may cause extrinsic alveolitis.

Previous chest radiographs

It is often vital to obtain a previous chest radiograph for comparison with recent films and the patient must be prompted to recall when and where he last had a radiograph. If it can be shown that a certain abnormality has been present for many years and is unaltered in appearance, it can usually be assumed that it is benign in nature and unnecessary investigations may be avoided.

FURTHER READING

Mason F, Swash M 1980 Hutchison's Clinical Methods, 17th edn. Cassell, London

4

Physical examination

The technique of physical examination is mastered by repeated practice at the bedside. This section outlines the method of examination of the respiratory system (Table 3) and describes abnormalities which may be detected at each stage of the examination. Physical examination always includes examination of the other systems.

Table 3 A guide for examination of the respiratory system

General examination	Dyspnoea
	Central cyanosis
	Finger clubbing
	Sputum
Upper respiratory tract	Ears, nose, teeth, tonsils, pharynx
Cervical and axillary lymph nodes	
Chest	
Inspection	Respiratory rate, rhythm, depth
	Shape and symmetry
	Movement
Palpation	Apex beat, trachea
	Expansion
	Vocal fremitus
Percussion	Resonance of percussion note
	Resistance to percussion
Auscultation	Quality of the breath sounds
	Intensity of the breath sounds
	Adventitious sounds
	Vocal resonance

The findings on each side of the chest are compared at each stage of the examination.

GENERAL EXAMINATION

The patient's general condition and appearance are observed before examining the chest. It is essential to look for dyspnoea and central cyanosis. It is then advisable to examine the hands for finger clubbing and to look inside the patient's sputum mug. These observations are of prime importance and may be forgotten if left until a later stage of the examination.

Cyanosis

Cyanosis is the name given to a dusky blue colour of the skin and mucous membranes due to the presence of increased amounts of reduced haemoglobin. There are two types of cyanosis.

Peripheral cyanosis

This is caused by sluggish blood flow through the peripheral parts of the body which allows increased extraction of oxygen from the capillary blood in the peripheral tissues. The oxygen saturation of the arterial blood is normal. Peripheral cyanosis affects the fingers, ears, cheeks, and the outer aspects of the lips. These parts are blue and often feel cold; warm well perfused regions like the tongue and the inside of the mouth are not affected. The effect of temperature is emphasized because cold produces peripheral vasoconstriction and is the commonest cause of peripheral cyanosis. Peripheral cyanosis is often seen on a cold morning or after swimming. Diseases which cause low cardiac output produce peripheral cyanosis as a result of poor peripheral circulation. Cardiac failure may cause peripheral cyanosis although more commonly it produces central cyanosis.

Central cyanosis

This is due to reduced oxygen saturation of the arterial blood. Central cyanosis is not clinically obvious until the arterial oxygen saturation falls below 80 per cent which corresponds to a P_aO_2 of less than 50 mmHg. Thus central cyanosis is a late sign of hypoxaemia. Central cyanosis may be visible in any part of the body, but in particular, warm well perfused areas like the tongue and the inside of the mouth are blue. Cyanosis of the tongue differentiates central from peripheral cyanosis. Central cyanosis is usually caused by respiratory or cardiac disease.

Respiratory disease. Reduced arterial oxygen saturation may occur in diseases such as pneumonia, pulmonary collapse, acute asthma, chronic bronchitis and emphysema and pulmonary embolism. The main mechanism responsible is ventilation-perfusion imbalance (p. 12).

Cardiac disease. Congenital heart diseases with a right to left shunt cause central cyanosis because venous blood passes directly into the systemic circulation without being oxygenated. Acute left ventricular failure may produce central cyanosis as a result of ventilation-perfusion imbalance. Oxygen therapy relieves cyanosis due to respiratory disease but does not improve cyanosis resulting from right to left shunts.

Polycythaemia. Central cyanosis is a feature of polycythaemia because the increased concentration of haemoglobin is accompanied by increased levels of reduced haemoglobin.

Finger clubbing

Finger clubbing is an important physical sign and is commonly due to respiratory disease. Finger clubbing is characterized by obliteration of the angle between the base of the nail and the skin on the dorsum of the terminal phalanx, and increased curvature of the nails in the longitudinal and transverse diameters (Fig. 6). These changes are best recognized by holding the patient's fingers level with the eyes and inspecting them from the side. As finger clubbing progresses, there is increase in the soft tissue of the ends of the fingers and they develop a drumstick shape. Occasionally severe clubbing is accompanied by pain and swelling of the joints of the hands, feet, wrists and ankles. This is called *hypertrophic pulmonary osteoarthropathy* and is usually due to bronchial carcinoma. Radiographs may

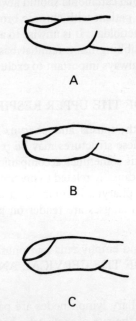

A

B

C

Fig. 6 Finger clubbing. a, Normal finger, b, Slight clubbing, c, Gross clubbing.

show subperiosteal new bone formation at the ends of the long bones near the wrist and ankle.

Finger clubbing causes increased nail bed fluctuation, a difficult physical sign. Finger clubbing is sometimes accompanied by clubbing of the toes.

The mechanism responsible for the development of clubbing is not known but in some cases it is related to the presence of sepsis. The causes of finger clubbing are shown in Table 4.

Table 4 Dieases associated with finger clubbing

Respiratory diseases	Cardiac diseases
Bronchial carcinoma	Cyanotic congenital heart disease
Bronchiectasis	Subacute bacterial endocarditis
Lung abscess	Abdominal diseases
Empyema	Ulcerative colitis
Fibrosing alveolitis	Cirrhosis of the liver
Asbestosis	Familial clubbing
Pleural fibroma	
Mesothelioma	
Tuberculosis	

Chronic bronchitis, emphysema and sarcoidosis do not cause finger clubbing. Bronchial carcinoma should always be suspected when clubbing is seen in a patient with chronic bronchitis since both diseases have the same aetiology. It is unwise to assume without further investigation that clubbing has a familial basis since familial clubbing is rare and it is always important to exclude underlying disease.

EXAMINATION OF THE UPPER RESPIRATORY TRACT

The ears, nose, teeth, tonsils and pharynx should be inspected, because disease of these structures may be related to disease of the chest. Allergic rhinitis sometimes accompanies asthma while severe dental caries may be causally related to pneumonia and lung abscess. Inflammation of the pharynx is common in upper respiratory tract infections. The nasal sinuses are tender on palpation in acute and chronic sinusitis.

EXAMINATION OF THE CERVICAL AND AXILLARY LYMPH NODES

The cervical and axillary lymph nodes are palpated systematically. They are sometimes the site of metastatic bronchial carcinoma and may be involved in tuberculosis and sarcoidosis.

EXAMINATION OF THE CHEST

The chest is examined by the time-honoured methods of inspection, palpation, percussion and auscultation. By these methods it is possible to detect signs caused by changes in the physical properties of the lungs and pleura. The position of a physical sign is correlated with the surface markings of the fissures of the lung which may help to localize it to one or more lobes (p. 2). Pleural effusion and pneumothorax give rise to signs which do not conform to a lobar distribution. It is essential that the chest is completely uncovered and the patient is kept warm. At each stage of the examination the right side of the chest is compared with the left.

Inspection

1. *Respiratory rate, rhythm* and *depth* are observed and it is noted whether the patient is using the accessory muscles of respiration and whether breathing causes pain.
2. *The shape and symmetry of the chest* are examined from front and behind. There are several different types of chest deformity:

   (a) *Harrison's sulcus.* This is a concave deformity of the lower ribs just above the costal margins and is usually the result of chronic asthma in childhood.

   (b) *Barrel shaped chest.* Increase in the anteroposterior diameter of the chest is a sign of hyperinflation and the chest may be barrel shaped in emphysema and during an acute attack of asthma.

   (c) *Funnel chest.* (Pectus excavatum) This funnel shaped depression of the lower end of the sternum is usually a congenital abnormality and it rarely causes symptoms.

   (d) *Pigeon chest.* (Pectus carinatum) This deformity is characterized by a sharp prominence of the upper part of the sternum. Pigeon chest is usually a congenital abnormality but it may develop in children with severe chronic asthma.

   (e) *Kyphoscoliosis.* Severe spinal deformity causes asymmetry of the chest wall and may occasionally cause breathlessness due to decreased vital capacity.

3. *The movement of the chest wall* is compared on each side. In health both sides of the chest move equally and this may be confirmed later by palpation. Reduced chest movement and flattening of the chest on one side indicate an abnormality on that side.

Reduced chest wall movement on one side may be due to the following:

Pulmonary collapse

Localized pulmonary fibrosis, e.g. bronchiectasis, tuberculosis
Pneumonic consolidation
Pleural effusion
Pneumothorax
Pain

Symmetrical reduction of chest wall movement indicates a diffuse abnormality:

Chronic bronchitis
Emphysema
Diffuse pulmonary fibrosis, e.g. fibrosing alveolitis

Intercostal indrawing is a feature of airways obstruction.

Palpation

1. The position of the apex beat and trachea

These are determined by palpation. Normally the apex beat lies in the 5th left intercostal space on the midclavicular line and the trachea lies centrally in the suprasternal notch. Cardiac failure causes displacement of the apex beat to the left but does not affect the position of the trachea.

Displacement of both the apex beat and trachea to the same side suggests that the position of the mediastinum has altered, either as a result of diseases which pull the mediastinum towards the affected side or those which push it away from the affected side. These are summarized as follows:

Deviation of the mediastinum towards the affected side:
Pulmonary collapse
Localized pulmonary fibrosis.

Deviation of the mediastinum away from the affected side:
Pleural effusion
Pneumothorax.

In practice displacement of the apex beat and especially the treachea is often difficult to detect. Tracheal deviation is obvious only when there is fibrosis or collapse of an upper lobe or collapse of the whole lung. Collapse or fibrosis of a lower lobe and a small effusion or pneumothorax do not cause detectable tracheal deviation.

2. Chest expansion

This is measured anteriorly and posteriorly by placing the hands symmetrically on each side of the chest. Chest expansion is normally about 5 cm and may be measured with a tape measure. The causes of reduced chest expansion have been discussed above.

3. Vocal fremitus

This is the name given to the vibrations which are felt on the chest wall when the patient speaks: usually the patient is asked to repeat a phrase such as '99' while each side of the chest is felt in turn with the same hand. Changes in vocal fremitus are usually difficult to detect and it is not an important chest sign. The causes of altered vocal fremitus are the same as those which affect vocal resonance (p. 42).

Percussion

The middle finger of the left hand is placed horizontally on the chest wall and the middle phalanx is struck sharply once or twice at right angles with the tip of the middle finger of the right hand. It is important to mould the left hand to the contour of the chest wall and to deliver the percussing stroke with a loose swinging action of the wrist.

Starting at the top of the chest corresponding areas on each side are percussed in turn. The front and back of the chest and the axillary regions are examined systematically. If possible percussion should be carried out with the patient sitting up.

The examiner must listen carefully to the resonance of the percussion note and feel for the degree of resistance to percussion. Both are affected by the thickness of the chest wall and by the different densities of the lungs, heart and liver. It is important to learn the normal limits of lung resonance and the contour of the cardiac dullness. *These are appreciated more readily by repeated examination of patients than by reading anatomical texts.* It is worth remembering that during quiet breathing the upper level of the liver dullness on the right is the 6th rib in the midclavicular line. If the chest is resonant below this level it is a sign of hyperinflation. This may be due to asthma or emphysema; in asthma the hyperinflation is transient and in emphysema it is permanent.

The percussion note over the lungs is affected by the volume of air in the lungs and the presence of air or fluid in the pleural cavity. 'Dullness' is the clinical term used to describe impairment of the percussion note. The causes of alteration of the percussion note are as follows:

Dullness on percussion:
   Pleural effusion—'stony dullness'
   Pneumonic consolidation
   Pulmonary collapse
   Localized pulmonary fibrosis.

Over a pleural effusion the percussion note is very dull and there is marked increase in the resistance to percussion. This finding is characteristic of effusion and is called 'stony dullness'. In pleural effusion the dullness extends in a semi-circle from the front to the back of the chest in contrast to pulmonary collapse and consolidation in which the impaired percussion note occurs over the affected lobe.

Hyper-resonant percussion note:

Pneumothorax

Emphysema

Auscultation

Auscultation is carried out systematically over corresponding areas on each side of the chest while the patient breathes fairly deeply with the mouth open. The following observations are made: the quality and intensity of the breath sounds, the presence or absence of adventitious sounds and the character of the vocal resonance. Vocal resonance is tested after the other examinations have been completed. A conscious effort must be made to concentrate upon each observation in turn, otherwise important abnormalities are overlooked; it is only too easy to be distracted by the patient in the next bed or by a pretty nurse!

1. The quality of breath sounds

There are two types of breath sounds, vesicular and bronchial. Bronchial breath sounds are not normally heard over the lungs.

Vesicular breath sounds are the normal sounds heard on auscultation of the chest and are produced by the movement of air in and out of the lungs. Vesicular breathing is rustling in quality. The inspiratory sound is louder than the expiratory sound; it is heard throughout inspiration and is followed immediately by the expiratory sound which is audible only during the earlier part of expiration. Prolonged expiration indicates airways obstruction, e.g., asthma, chronic bronchitis and emphysema.

Bronchial breath sounds (bronchial breathing) are blowing in quality, the duration of expiration is as long or longer than inspiration, the intensity and pitch of the expiratory sound is higher than that of the inspiratory sound and sometimes a short gap is noticeable between inspiration and expiration. Such a definition has little practical value and there is no substitute for listening repeatedly to a patient with bronchial breathing. Once learnt the sign is never forgotten. It is said that bronchial breathing is similar to the sound heard by listening over the trachea, but this is a poor analogy. The breath sounds normally heard between the scapulae and over the right upper zone anteriorly are sometimes rather bronchial in quality because of the proximity of the trachea and main bronchi.

Bronchial breathing occurs when the sounds produced by the movement of air through the trachea and large bronchi are transmitted directly to the chest wall by abnormalities of the lung or pleura which act as good conducting media for these sounds but prevent the normal movement of air through the alveoli.

Bronchial breathing occurs in the following conditions:

Common: Pneumonic consolidation
            At the top of a pleural effusion
Uncommon: Pulmonary collapse
            Localized pulmonary fibrosis
            Pneumothorax
            Large lung cavities, e.g. tuberculosis.

Bronchial breathing heard over a large cavity is similar to the sound produced by blowing across the top of a bottle and is sometimes termed amphoric or cavernous breathing.

2. The intensity of the breath sounds

The intensity of the breath sounds is reduced by conditions which reduce the entry of air to the lung or prevent conduction of the breath sounds to the chest wall. The degree to which the breath sounds are reduced depends upon the extent of the underlying lesion; they may be slightly or moderately reduced in intensity or they may be absent.

Reduced intensity of the breath sounds:
    Pulmonary collapse
    Localized pulmonary fibrosis
    Pneumonia—Lobar consolidation or bronchopneumonia
    Emphysema
    Neoplasm
    Pleural effusion
    Pneumothorax.

3. Adventitious sounds

These are of three types, crepitations, rhonchi and pleural rub.

Crepitations are bubbling or crackling sounds similar to the noise heard when hairs next to the ear are rubbed together. Crepitations are discontinuous and are heard mainly at the end of deep inspiration and the beginning of expiration. They are caused by the opening up of alveoli or bronchioles containing secretions, by the separation of thickened alveolar walls or by the movement of air through bronchioles or bronchi containing secretions.

Crepitations commonly occur in the following diseases:
  Pneumonia
  Bronchiectasis
  Cardiac failure
  Allergic alveolitis
  Fibrosing alveolitis.

Crepitations may be fine or coarse in quality. Fine crepitations are often heard in cardiac failure and coarse crepitations in bronchiectasis, but it is unreliable to attempt diagnosis merely upon the quality of the crepitations. In allergic alveolitis and fibrosing alveolitis the crepitations have a peculiar dry crackling quality and are sometimes termed 'dry' crepitations. Crepitations are sometimes called râles.

Rhonchi are continuous high, medium or low pitched sounds produced by air flowing through narrowed bronchi. High pitched rhonchi are whistling in quality and are produced in the smaller bronchi; low pitched, sonorous rhonchi arise from the larger bronchi. Rhonchi are heard when the patient has wheeze and are the result of airways obstruction by excessive secretions, mucosal oedema or muscle spasm. Rhonchi are usually a sign of asthma or chronic bronchitis and emphysema but occasionally localized rhonchi are heard over a bronchus which is partly occluded by a plug of mucus, tumour or foreign body. Rhonchi are louder during expiration than inspiration due to the normal expiratory narrowing of the bronchial tree. For the same reason, rhonchi are accentuated by forced expiration and this manoeuvre may be helpful in confirming their presence in a doubtful case. Expiration is prolonged in airways obstruction to compensate for the obstruction to air flow. Low pitched rhonchi due to secretions in large bronchi may be confused with coarse crepitations but will often disappear after coughing.

Pleural rub is a creaking sound caused by inflamed pleural surfaces rubbing together during breathing. The sound is heard during corresponding phases of inspiration and expiration and becomes louder on deep breathing or if the stethoscope is pressed hard against the chest. Pleural rub may be confused with coarse crepitations or localized low pitched rhonchi, but the latter often disappear if the patient is asked to cough. Pleural rub is a sign of pleurisy which is usually secondary to pneumonia or pulmonary infarction. Pleural rub is commonly accompanied by pleuritic pain in the same region.

4. Vocal resonance
This is elicited by asking the patient to say '99' in a deep voice while listening to the chest. The factors which give rise to bronchial

breathing may cause increased vocal resonance and sometimes increased vocal fremitus. The commonest cause is pneumonic consolidation and the main value of vocal resonance is to confirm the presence of bronchial breathing in such cases. Often conduction is increased to such a degree that when the patient whispers '22' it sounds as though it is being whispered directly into the examiner's ear. This is called *whispering pectoriloquy*.

The physical findings are correlated after the examination and an attempt is made to deduce the underlying pathological process. Certain pathological changes in the lungs and pleura give rise to characteristic groups of signs but these are obvious only when the lesion is extensive (Table 5).

Table 5 Summary of the main physical signs in some common disorders.

	Movement of chest wall	Media-stinal dis-placement	Percussion note	Breath sounds	Adven-titious sounds
Pneumonic consolidation	Reduced	Nil	Dull	Bronchial	Crepit-ations
Pulmonary collapse	Reduced	Towards affected side	Dull	Reduced or absent vesicular*	Nil
Localized fibrosis	Reduced	Towards affected side	Dull	Vesicular*	Crepit-ations
Pleural effusion	Reduced	Away from affected side	Stony dull	Reduced or absent†	Nil
Pneumothorax	Reduced	Away from affected side	Hyper-resonant	Reduced or absent vesicular*	Nil

*Bronchial breathing is occasionally present.
†Bronchial at the top of the effusion.

CLINICAL DIAGNOSIS

Diagnosis is a reasoning process which correlates the information obtained from the history and the physical examination.

The patient's age is a primary consideration in diagnosis since some diseases occur predominantly in certain age groups. For example, bronchial carcinoma, chronic bronchitis and thrombo-embolism mainly affect patients over the age of 40.

The duration of the illness is also important. Diseases such as pneumonia and pulmonary infarction cause acute illness, while tuberculosis usually presents as a chronic illness. Bronchial carcinoma tends to give rise to persistent symptoms.

The first stage in diagnosis is to review the patient's history. The presenting symptoms are evaluated in turn and thought is given to the possible anatomical, physiological and pathological basis of each symptom. It is often helpful to write down the possible causes of each symptom. Attention is then paid to the relationship between symptoms. Certain combinations of symptoms are sometimes sufficiently characteristic to provide an accurate provisional diagnosis. For example, haemoptysis, pleuritic pain and breathlessness of sudden onset are very suggestive of pulmonary infarction.

The past history, family history, occupational history and social history are then reviewed and relevant information, e.g. family history of or exposure to tuberculosis, pets, dust exposure, cigarette smoking, overseas travel, is correlated with the presenting symptoms. A differential diagnosis is drawn up which includes conditions which are probable or possible causes of the patient's illness.

The second stage in diagnosis is to review the results of the physical examination. Examination may have revealed signs which are sufficiently distinctive to allow a pathological diagnosis, e.g. consolidation, collapse, airways obstruction, pneumothorax or effusion.

The third stage in diagnosis is to correlate the physical findings with the patient's symptoms, and modify the existing differential diagnosis. The most likely cause of the symptoms and signs is selected as the provisional diagnosis.

The final diagnosis is sometimes only obtained after consideration of the results of relevant investigations.

FURTHER READING

Mason F, Swash M 1980 Hutchison's clinical methods, 17th Edn. Cassell, London
Macleod J G 1979 Clinical examination, 5th Edn. Churchill Livingstone, Edinburgh

5

Investigation of the respiratory system

The investigations which are carried out in a particular patient are determined by the clinical findings, and if sufficient thought is given to their selection it is usually easy to confirm the clinical diagnosis.

RADIOGRAPHIC EXAMINATION

Chest radiograph

The chest radiograph is the most valuable investigation in respiratory medicine. It reveals abnormalities which cannot be detected by physical examination and excludes certain serious diseases. If the radiograph is normal it is most unlikely that the patient has pneumonia, pulmonary tuberculosis, bronchial carcinoma, pulmonary sarcoidosis or pneumoconiosis. A chest radiograph should be taken of any patient with respiratory symptoms unless they are trivial or transient. Mass radiography can be used to screen populations for tuberculosis (p. 200).

It is essential to become familiar with the appearances of the normal chest radiograph and of the common abnormalities, and the student must avoid the bad habit of reading the radiologist's report without seeing the films. The physician should feel personally responsible for viewing his patients' radiographs.

The standard radiograph is a postero-anterior (PA) view and is taken with the X-ray tube behind the patient and the cassette against the front of the patient's chest. An antero-posterior (AP) view or portable film is taken when the patient is confined to bed. The X-ray tube is then positioned in front of the patient and the cassette is placed against the patient's back. This means that the heart is further from the plate than in a PA film and the diverging rays magnify the size of the heart. For this reason it is not possible to give an accurate assessment of heart size in an AP film.

Before reading a chest radiograph it is essential to check the following points:

1. The name on the radiograph; to make sure that it belongs to the correct patient.

2. The date on the radiograph.

3. Whether the radiograph is a PA or AP film; this can only be learnt by enquiry unless the film is marked 'portable'.

4. Which is the right side of the patient's chest and which is the left; markers on radiographs cannot be relied upon because they are sometimes placed on the wrong side. Normally the right hemidiaphragm is higher than the left; the aortic knuckle and heart lie predominantly on the left and gas in the stomach shows as a translucency under the left hemidiaphragm. The latter is the most reliable guide.

5. That the radiograph is 'centred'. The medial end of each clavicle should be equidistant from the spines of the vertebrae. These distances will not be equal if the patient's chest was turned to one side when the radiograph was taken. Rotation causes undue prominence of the mediastinum on the side opposite to which the patient was turned and this must be allowed for in the interpretation of hilar and mediastinal shadows.

Examination of the PA radiograph

Examination must be systematic otherwise abnormalities are overlooked. The following structures are examined in turn and at each stage the right side is carefully compared with the left:

Trachea	Lung fields
Upper mediastinum and aorta	Gastric air bubble
Hila of the lungs	Subdiaphragmatic areas
Heart size and borders	Soft tissues
Diaphragm	Bony skeleton
Cardiophrenic and costophrenic angles	

Such detailed examination may seem unnecessary but it is surprising how often the clue to correct diagnosis does not lie in the lung fields but in other thoracic structures. For example, a pulmonary opacity can be assumed to be neoplastic if the radiograph also shows an osteolytic lesion in one of the ribs. Particular attention is paid to the heart shadow because a collapsed left lower lobe or a large hiatus hernia appears as a shadow behind the heart.

Lung zones

The lung fields are divided into lung zones.

The *upper zone* extends from the top of the lung to a horizontal line drawn through the lower border of the anterior end of the 2nd rib.

The *mid zone* extends from the lower border of the upper zone to a horizontal line drawn through the lower border of the anterior end of the 4th rib.

The *lower zone* extends from the lower border of the mid zone to the hemidiaphragm.

The position of an abnormality in the lung fields is described in relation to the lung zones because it is sometimes impossible to localize its anatomical position in the PA film. A shadow in the right mid zone may lie in the upper, middle or lower lobe. A lateral radiograph is used for exact anatomical diagnosis; it also reveals lesions which lie behind the heart. A lordotic radiograph (apical view) provides a good view of the lung apices.

Simple terms such as 'mottling', 'shadow', or 'opacity' are used to describe abnormalities in the lung fields. In many cases it is unwise to attempt a precise pathological diagnosis from the radiograph alone. For accurate diagnosis, the radiograph findings must be correlated with the *patient's age*, the *symptoms and signs* and the *results of other investigations*.

The following radiographic abnormalities are common diagnostic problems:

1. Ill defined, localized, non homogeneous opacity, e.g. lobular pneumonia, pulmonary infarction, tuberculosis, bronchial carcinoma.
2. Homogeneous opacity, e.g. lobar pneumonia, pulmonary collapse, pleural effusion.
3. Solitary circumscribed opacity or 'coin' lesion, e.g. bronchial carcinoma, tuberculoma, benign tumour.
4. Solitary cavitated opacity, e.g. bronchial carcinoma, lung abscess, tuberculosis.
5. Hilar opacity, e.g. bronchial carcinoma, sarcoid, lymphoma.
6. Mediastinal opacity, e.g. mediastinal tumours.
7. Diffuse radiographic opacities, which may be miliary, nodular, reticular or reticulo-nodular in appearance. The term 'miliary mottling' is given to multiple diffuse opacities which measure 2 mm or less in diameter, e.g. miliary tuberculosis, sarcoidosis. Nodular opacities measure 3 to 10 mm in diameter, e.g. bronchopneumonia, pneumoconiosis. Reticular abnormalities consist of a network of linear opacities which sometimes form a honeycomb pattern, e.g. fibrosing alveolitis.

These abnormalities are illustrated diagramatically in subsequent chapters.

Sometimes the interlobar fissures of the lung are visible. In the PA film the horizontal fissure appears as a fine horizontal line at the level of the 4th costal cartilage. The oblique fissure is not visible in the PA view but is sometimes seen in the lateral film. It begins at the level of the 5th thoracic vertebra and runs downwards and forwards to meet the diaphragm at the junction of its anterior and middle thirds. Fibrosis or collapse of the lung causes displacement of the fissures. Occasionally accessory fissures are present of which the commonest is the azygos fissure. This appears as a curved line running downwards and medially from the apex of the right lung to the azygos vein which lies above the right hilum. It is a developmental anomaly which occurs in about 1 per cent of people. The lung medial to the fissure is part of the right upper lobe and is called the azygos lobe. It has no clinical significance.

Tomography
Tomograms are radiographs of serial sections of the lung and are used to obtain clearer definition of abnormalities seen in the PA film. Cavities and calcification are best demonstrated by tomography. These findings always suggest the possibility of tuberculosis but they may also occur in bronchial carcinoma and other diseases. Tomograms may be helpful in the diagnosis of hilar enlargement, circumscribed pulmonary lesions ('coin' lesions p. 177) and vascular abnormalities.

Screening of the diaphragm
Diaphragmatic movement is visualized during fluoroscopic screening. Paradoxical movement of a hemidiaphragm indicates diaphragmatic paralysis. This is usually due to involvement of the phrenic nerve at the hilum by bronchial carcinoma.

Bronchography
If radiopaque medium is instilled into the trachea and bronchi under local or general anaesthesia, radiographs will show the outline of the bronchial tree. Bronchography is used to confirm the presence and extent of bronchiectasis prior to surgery (p. 110).

Barium swallow
Barium swallow is used to detect oesophageal compression by mediastinal tumours and metastases (p. 174). Occasionally barium swallow provides diagnostic information in recurrent pneumonia which is secondary to aspiration of food from an oesophageal stricture or carcinoma.

Pulmonary scanning
Macroaggregated albumin labelled with technetium 99 m is injected

intravenously and the aggregates become temporarily trapped in the pulmonary arteriolar-capillary bed where they emit gamma rays which are detected by scanning the chest. The intensity of radio-active emission gives an indication of pulmonary perfusion and the technique is used to detect obstruction of blood flow by pulmonary emboli. Perfusion defects also occur in chronic bronchitis, asthma, emphysema, pneumonia and bronchial carcinoma and the results of scanning must be correlated with the clinical findings and the chest radiograph. This technique is most useful in the diagnosis of suspected pulmonary embolism when the chest radiograph is normal (p. 157). When other pulmonary pathology is present a ventilation scan (Xenon[33]) is necessary for interpretation of the perfusion scan.

Isotope scanning of the liver, brain and bones is often part of the preoperative investigation of bronchial carcinoma.

Pulmonary angiography

Radiopaque medium injected through a catheter into the pulmonary artery will outline the pulmonary circulation. Pulmonary angiography is mainly used to detect congenital anomalies of the pulmonary circulation and is sometimes used for the diagnosis of pulmonary embolism.

Other techniques

The role of computerised axial tomography in respiratory medicine is not yet clear. Ultra-sound is useful for localising pockets of pleural fluid and hepatic metastases.

PERIPHERAL BLOOD EXAMINATION

Estimation of the haemoglobin, the total and differential white cell count and erythrocyte sedimentation rate is a routine procedure in most patients with persistent symptoms although in respiratory medicine the results are of limited diagnostic value.

Anaemia is uncommon in respiratory diseases except in tuberculosis, severe pneumonia and extensive malignancy.

Polycythaemia sometimes develops in conditions characterized by chronic hypoxaemia but is not a constant finding. It can be differentiated from polycythaemia rubra vera by the normal white cell count and platelet count.

Leucocytosis of mild to moderate degree, 12 000 to 16 000/mm^3, occurs in about 80 per cent of patients with pneumonia and in about 20 per cent of patients with tuberculosis and pulmonary infarction. Leucocytosis is relatively uncommon in chronic bronchitis and bronchiectasis. Leucopenia may occur in fulminating pneumonia.

Eosinophilia occurs in asthma and extremely high eosinophil counts are common in pulmonary eosinophilia (p. 245).

The ESR is elevated in about 80 per cent of patients with pneumonia but is frequently normal in other infections, including tuberculosis, and in bronchial carcinoma. A very high ESR is common in collagen disorders and multiple myeloma, diseases which sometimes affect the respiratory system.

SPUTUM EXAMINATION

It is important that the specimen collected for examination is sputum and not saliva; sometimes an adequate specimen may only be obtained after chest physiotheraphy. The macroscopic appearance of the sputum is recorded before proceeding to detailed examination.

Bacteria
Bacteriological examination of the sputum is important in the diagnosis and management of acute respiratory infections. Sputum should be collected before starting antibiotic treatment and examined as soon as possible after collection.

Sputum smears stained with Gram stain may provide information which is of immediate diagnostic help, especially in a desperately ill patient; demonstration of bacteria resembling staphylococci influences the choice of antibiotic treatment.

Sputum culture takes 24 hours. Interpretation of the results is sometimes difficult since isolation of a particular organism is no proof that it is the causal agent. Isolation in heavy growth is more significant than isolation of a few colonies. Gram negative bacteria are frequently isolated after a patient has started antibiotic therapy but they are then rarely aetiologically significant.

Pharyngeal swabs may be examined if the patient is unable to cough up sputum, but the results are difficult to interpret because 40 per cent of healthy people carry staphylococci and pneumococci in the nasopharynx. Transtracheal aspiration may yield useful specimens.

Sensitivity tests are carried out on bacteria isolated from sputum culture.

M. tuberculosis
Examination for tubercle bacilli should be carried out in all patients in whom the clinical or radiographic findings could be due to tuberculosis. This includes all patients with pneumonia.

Sputum smears stained by the Ziehl-Neelsen method are examined microscopically for acid-fast bacteria.

Sputum culture is necessary to confirm that acid-fast bacteria are *M. tuberculosis* Sputum culture takes 3 to 6 weeks and sensitivity tests take a further 4 weeks. It is usual to send three sputum specimens for examination for tubercle bacilli. If no sputum is available, laryngeal swabs or gastric washings are examined. A positive Ziehl-Neelsen stain obtained from gastric washings may be due to saphrophytic acid-fast bacteria and should be interpreted with caution.

Viruses, M. pneumoniae, Legionella pneumophila
Sputum, nasal washings and pharyngeal swabs from patients with acute respiratory infections can be cultured for viruses, *M. pneumoniae* and *L pneumophila* but isolation rates are low.

Fungi
Sputum culture for fungi is occasionally helpful. Fungi may cause pneumonia in patients with immunological disorders and *Aspergillus fumigatus* is sometimes responsible for asthma, e.g. allergic bronchopulmonary aspergillosis.

Pus cells
Pus cells may be seen in the Gram film in acute bacterial infections and the number of pus cells correlates well with the severity of the infection.

Eosinophils
Eosinophils are often present in the sputum in large numbers in bronchial asthma and allergic bronchopulmonary aspergillosis. They can be identified in a Leishman stained sputum smear.

Malignant cells
Sputum cytology is a valuable diagnostic investigation and malignant cells can be demonstrated in sputum in 80 per cent of patients with bronchial carcinoma. False positive results are rare. At least three specimens of sputum are examined: the fresher the specimen the better the diagnostic yield.

Asbestos bodies
Asbestos bodies may be present in sputum smears from asbestos workers and indicate exposure to asbestos. They do not signify the presence of asbestosis.

The physician will invariably gain valuable diagnostic and therapeutic advice by personally discussing the results of sputum examinations with the bacteriologist and pathologist.

SEROLOGICAL TESTS

Infection

Complement fixation tests are useful in diagnosing some infections. Specimens of serum taken at the onset of the illness and 10 to 14 days later are examined for antibodies against the following antigens: influenza, parainfluenza, adenovirus, respiratory syncytial virus, psittacosis, *R. burneti, M.pneumoniae, L. pneumophila* and *Pneumocystis carinii*. A fourfold rise in antibody titre indicates a recent infection. Serum is also examined for cold agglutinins which are frequently present in, but not specific to, mycoplasmal infections.

Allergic alveolitis

In some types of allergic alveolitis the diagnosis may be confirmed by the demonstration of precipitating antibodies against the causal antigen (p. 217).

TUBERCULIN TEST

The tuberculin skin test is a useful diagnostic aid in tuberculosis and is discussed in detail on page 186.

KVEIM TEST

The Kveim test is positive in 70–80 per cent of patients with sarcoidosis (p. 209). An intradermal injection of a suspension of human sarcoid extract produces a nodule at the injection site and biopsy 4 to 6 weeks after the injection shows sarcoid tissue. The Kveim test is of most help in patients with bilateral hilar lymphadenopathy or diffuse pulmonary abnormalities.

ELECTROCARDIOGRAPHY

The ECG is helpful in differentiating pain due to myocardial infarction from pain due to respiratory disease. Evidence of right heart strain is common in the later stages of chronic bronchitis emphysema and is sometimes present in pulmonary embolism.

BRONCHOSCOPY

The trachea, main bronchi and the orifices of the lobar and segmental bronchi may be seen through a bronchoscope. The rigid bronchoscope is an illuminated metal tube which is passed through the mouth into the bronchial tree. Bronchoscopy is carried out under local or general anaesthesia. Fibreoptic bronchoscopes are flexible and thinner and permit examination of subsegmental bronchi and beyond. Bronchoscopy is particularly valuable in the diagnosis of bronchial carcinoma and over 60 per cent of tumours are visible. At bronchoscopy a biopsy may be taken for histological study and bronchial secretions collected for examination for malignant cells and tubercle bacilli.

Bronchoscopy is indicated in the following situations:

Suspected bronchial carcinoma
Haemoptysis
Stridor
Inhaled foreign body
Obstruction of the bronchial tree by excessive secretions.

PLEURAL ASPIRATION AND BIOPSY

Pleural aspiration is an essential diagnostic and therapeutic procedure in pleural effusion (p. 230). The following studies are carried out on the pleural fluid: cell count, including examination for malignant cells; estimation of specific gravity, protein and sugar content; culture for bacteria including tubercle bacilli.

Needle biopsy of the parietal pleura provides a histological diagnosis in about 60 per cent of tuberculous and malignant effusions. Pleural biopsy should not be attempted in the absence of pleural effusion because it may cause pulmonary haemorrhage.

SCALENE NODE BIOPSY

Biopsy of the scalene lymph nodes provides a histological diagnosis in sarcoidosis, but is often unnecessary because the diagnosis can be made on clinical grounds or by a Kveim test. In suspected bronchial carcinoma this procedure may establish the diagnosis if a palpable node is biopsied, but blind biopsy of the scalene nodes is rarely positive.

MEDIASTINOSCOPY

Mediastinal lymph nodes may be biopsied using a mediastinoscope which is inserted through an incision in the suprasternal notch and passed downwards through the pretracheal fascia to the upper mediastinum. Mediastinoscopy is used preoperatively to determine whether bronchial carcinoma has spread to the mediastinal nodes. It is sometimes useful in the investigation of a hilar mass.

LUNG BIOPSY

Lung biopsy is sometimes indicated in diffuse lung disease and maybe carried out perentaneously (high speed drill, Tru-cut needle, Nordenstrom screw needle),transbronchially via the fibreoptic bronchoscope, or by thoracotomy (open lung biopsy). Lung biopsy should not be undertaken lightly because of the risk of pulmonary bleeding and it can often be avoided by careful clinical reasoning and the use of appropriate investigations.

PULMONARY FUNCTION TESTS

Pulmonary function tests are discussed in Chapter 1.

Other investigations which are sometimes useful include skin tests in asthma (p. 121), serum protein electrophoresis in multiple myeloma and immune deficiency states (p. 76), and estimations of antinuclear factor and rheumatoid factor in collagen disorders.

FURTHER READING

Clark T J H 1981 Clinical investigation of respiratory disease. Chapman and Hall, London

Cruickshank R 1973 Medical microbiology, 12th Edn. Churchill Livingstone, Edinburgh

Fraser R G, Pare J A P 1979 Diagnosis of diseases of the chest, 2nd Edn. Saunders, Philadelphia

Le Roux B T, Dodds T C 1968 A second portfolio of chest radiographs. E & S Livingstone, Edinburgh

Stradling P 1981 Diagnostic bronchoscopy, 4th Edn. Churchill Livingstone, Edinburgh

6

Principles of treatment

MAINTAIN A CLEAR AIRWAY

The first principle in the treatment of respiratory disease is to maintain the patency of the patient's airway at all times. All other forms of treatment are secondary, since they will be ineffective if the patient is asphyxiated by retained secretions. The bronchial tree is most likely to be occluded by secretions in pneumonia, acute asthma and exacerbations of chronic bronchitis.

Respiratory failure can often be prevented if the physiotherapist and nursing staff regularly assist the patient to cough up secretions. Adequate fluids prevent dehydration and reduce sputum viscosity, facilitating expectoration. Sticky tenacious sputum is an ominous sign which indicates that hydration is inadequate.

If assisted coughing fails to keep the airway clear, it is necessary to carry out tracheobronchial suction. This may be done during laryngoscopy or bronchoscopy, or through an endotracheal tube which is passed through the mouth into the larynx and upper trachea. Intubation is essential when repeated suction is necessary; it also provides a means by which oxygen can be delivered directly into the trachea. A cuff on the endotracheal tube prevents inhalation of vomitus or secretions from the upper respiratory tract into the lungs. If assisted ventilation becomes necessary the endotracheal tube may be connected to a ventilator. Tracheostomy is carried out if tracheo-bronchial suction or assisted ventilation is required for more than a few days because prolonged intubation may cause ulceration of the trachea. Tracheostomy has the added advantage of reducing the dead space.

OXYGEN THERAPY

Indications for treatment
The main indication for oxygen therapy is hypoxaemia. Cotes has emphasised that during an acute respiratory illness oxygen should

be given immediately if $P_a O_2$ is less than 50 mmHg. It is also often advisable to administer oxygen to patients with less severe hypoxaemia. If the patient has central cyanosis severe hypoxaemia is present. Lesser degrees of hypoxaemia cannot be detected clinically but can often be assumed to be present in severe pneumonia, acute asthma and during an exacerbation of chronic bronchitis.

Patients with hypercapnia lose their normal responsiveness to carbon dioxide and depend on hypoxaemia for ventilatory drive. This mainly occurs in severe chronic bronchitis, and although treatment with high concentrations of oxygen relieves the hypoxaemia it removes the stimulus to respiration causing depression of ventilation and increase in $P_a CO_2$. This is avoided by giving oxygen in low concentrations, 24 to 28 per cent.

For these reasons blood gas analysis is often carried out before starting oxygen therapy, and it may also be necessary to monitor the blood gases during treatment. Despite the possible dangers of high concentrations of oxygen it is wrong to delay treatment while waiting for the results of blood gas analysis. In practice the rule is to give oxygen immediately if the patient has hypoxaemia or if this is suspected; giving low concentrations of oxygen with a Ventimask if the patient has chronic bronchitis or possible hypercapnia. The aim of oxygen therapy is to raise the $P_a O_2$ to at least 50 mmHg and preferably above 65 mmHg. In patients with hypercapnia assisted ventilation may be necessary if controlled oxygen therapy cannot achieve a $P_a O_2$ of 40 mmHg without depressing the pH below 7.25.

Methods of oxygen administration.
When ordering oxygen the method of administration, the concentration of inspired oxygen, the flow rate and the humidification must be specified.

Ventimask (Oxygenaire Ltd.). This mask employs the venturi principle to mix oxygen with air in constant proportions. The concentration of inspired oxygen is accurately controlled by using Ventimasks specifically designed to deliver 24, 28 or 35 per cent oxygen. Oxygen flow rates of 2 1/min, 41 1/min and 8 1/min respectively will provide these concentrations. A Ventimask is the best method of delivering oxygen to patients with chronic bronchitis and hypercapnia. Treatment is started with a 24 per cent mask but this is changed for a 28 per cent mask if the $P_a O_2$ remains below 50 mmHg, provided the increased inspired oxygen concentration does not cause more than 5 mm or so rise in $P_a CO_2$. Ventimasks have the added advantage that the oxygen does not require humidification because they deliver a high proportion of air.

Edinburgh mask (British Oxygen Co. Ltd.). This mask delivers 22 to 40 per cent oxygen using flow rates of 0.5 to 3 l/min. The Edinburgh mask may be used to treat patients with chronic bronchitis and hypercapnia, but the concentration of inspired oxygen is more difficult to control than with the Ventimask.

Nasal catheter. Catheters deliver approximately 25 to 40 per cent oxygen at flow rates of 2 to 6 l/min. The concentration of inspired oxygen is related to the flow rate and is difficult to control. Another disadvantage of nasal catheters is that the oxygen must be humidified. Nasal catheters have the advantage that they prevent rebreathing of carbon dioxide and do not interfere with eating. They are used when it is unnecessary to control accurately the inspired oxygen concentration and should not be used if hypercapnia is present.

Polymask (British Oxygen Co. Ltd). This type of mask delivers about 60 per cent oxygen using a flow rate of 6 l/min. They are used when high concentrations of oxygen are required but should not be used if the $P_a CO_2$ is raised. It is necessary to humidify the oxygen and small amounts of expired carbon dioxide may be rebreathed because the mask fits tightly over the face.

Oxygen tent. These supply 60 per cent oxygen at flow rates of 10 l/min but are seldom used because they interfere with patient care.

Mechanical ventilators may be used to supply oxygen but it is doubtful whether they have any advantages over other methods unless the patient requires assisted ventilation.

Emergency treatment. Mouth to mouth respiration or ventilation with an Ambu bag can be life saving in an emergency.

Domiciliary oxygen. An oxygen supply in the home is sometimes helpful to patients whose mobility is severely restricted by chronic lung disease. The oxygen may be supplied from a cylinder or an oxygen concentrator, and the patient is given a mask which will deliver a suitable concentration of oxygen. He must be instructed about flow rates and be warned about the risk of fire.

Dangers of oxygen therapy

Apart from the risk of aggravating hypercapnia, oxygen therapy may cause other complications. The lung may be damaged if concentrations of more than 40 per cent are given for more than 12 hours. In the neonatal period high concentrations of oxygen may cause retrolental fibroplasia.

ANTIBIOTIC THERAPY

Indications for treatment

Exacerbations of chronic bronchitis and emphysema, acute bronchitis and pneumonia are the commonest acute respiratory infections treated with antibiotics. Antibiotics are also frequently used in acute asthma because infection is often the precipitating factor.

Before starting treatment

A specimen of sputum is sent to the laboratory for Gram stain, bacterial culture and sensitivity tests before beginning treatment. In pneumonia it is also advisable to carry out blood culture. Antibiotics should be started before the results of sputum culture are available but it is sometimes helpful to examine the Gram stain before beginning treatment. If this shows cocci resembling staphylococci and the patient is moderately or severely ill it is probable that staphylococci are the causal organisms. It is then advisable to use an antibiotic which is effective against penicillin resistant staphylococci because a high proportion of staphylococci are resistant to penicillin. In life-threatening pneumonia appropriate antibiotics should not be withheld because of difficulty in obtaining sputum.

Choice of antibiotic

This depends upon the causal bacteria, but these can be predicted with a high degree of accuracy in most acute lower respiratory infections. Pneumonia is usually caused by *Str. pneumoniae* which is invariably sensitive to penicillin and ampicillin, and these are the antibiotics of choice. Acute bronchitis and exacerbations of chronic bronchitis are mainly caused by *Str. pneumoniae* or *H. influenzae*. Ampicillin is the antibiotic of choice in bronchitis because *H. influenzae* is sometimes resistant to penicillin.

Before beginning treatment it is essential to ask the patient whether he is allergic to penicillin or ampicillin, or has ever developed a rash or fever when treated with these drugs. If so, tetracycline, co-trimoxazole or erythromycin are effective substitutes. Cotrimoxazole is a combination of trimethoprim and sulphamethoxazole. In pneumonia penicillin is initially given by intramuscular injection but the other antibiotics are given by mouth unless the patient is desperately ill, when it may be necessary to use the intramuscular or intravenous routes. Side effects from the penicillins are uncommon with the exception of hypersensitivity which causes rash and fever on the 7th to 10th days of treatment. Ampicillin may cause diarrhoea.

Infections caused by *Staph. aureus* are treated with flucloxacillin, fusidic acid or methicillin if the organism is penicillin resistant, because these antibiotics are effective against penicillinase producing staphylococci.

These antibiotics are more effective against penicillin-resistant staphylococci when given in combination with benzyl penicillin. Benzyl penicillin is given alone if the staphylococci are known to be penicillin-sensitive.

Antibiotics effective in the treatment of infections due to other organisms are shown in Table 6. Gram negative bacteria such as *E. coli*, *Proteus* and *Pseudomonas* have not been included because they are rare causal agents of respiratory infections, although they may be isolated from sputum in patients receiving antibiotics. These bac-

Table 6 A guide to antibiotic therapy in acute respiratory infections

Aetiological agent	Antibiotic of choice	Adult dose	Usual route	Alternative antibiotic
Str. pneumoniae	Benzyl penicillin or	1 mega unit bd	i.m.	Tetracycline Co-trimoxazole
	Ampicillin	250 mg 6 hourly	Oral	Erythromycin
Staph. aureus	Benzyl penicillin (if sensitive) or	1 mega unit 6 hourly	i.m.	
	Flucloxacillin +	250–500 mg 4 to 6 hourly	Oral	Methicillin, Fusidic acid
	Benzyl penicillin (if penicillin resistant)		i.m. i.v.	Cephaloridine Erythromycin
H. influenzae	Ampicillin or Tetracycline	250 mg 6 hourly	Oral	Erythromycin Co-trimoxazole Benzyl penicillin + streptomycin
K. pneumoniae	Gentamicin + Chloramphenicol	80 mg 8 hourly + 500 mg 6 hourly	i.m. i.v. i.v.	Kanamycin
M. pneumoniae	Tetracycline	500 mg 6 hourly	Oral	Erythromycin
C. psittaci	Tetracycline	500 mg 6 hourly	Oral	Erythromycin
R. burneti	Tetracycline	500 mg 6 hourly	Oral	Erythromycin
L. pneumophila	Erythromycin	500 mg 6 hourly	Oral i.v.	Tetracycline

teria rarely require treatment but when necessary the results of sensitivity tests should be used as a guide for selection of the appropriate antibiotic. The bacteriologist will give helpful advice with this problem. Antibiotics effective against these Gram negative bacteria include gentamicin, carbenicillin, kanamycin, azlocillin, tobramycin, cefuroxime.

Signs of response to treatment.

These include improvement in clinical condition, fall in temperature, clearance of bacteria and pus from the sputum, and in pneumonia, resolution of the radiographic abnormalities. Usually the patient is afebrile and feels and looks better after 3 to 4 days. Antibiotic treatment should be continued for at least one week but longer treatment is often given in pneumonia.

Errors in treatment.

The main errors in chemotherapy are to stop treatment too soon or to change treatment unnecessarily. In most cases, penicillin, ampicillin or tetracycline are highly effective and to use new and powerful antibiotics without good reason will lead to an increase in resistant organisms.

BRONCHODILATOR THERAPY

Indications for treatment.

Bronchodilator drugs are used to relieve airways obstruction in asthma and chronic bronchitis. There are numerous bronchodilator preparations and Table 7 shows those in common use. Individual patient response is variable and measurement of FEV_1, FVC and/or PEFR before and after different bronchodilators provides a rational guide for the selection of an effective preparation for long term treatment (p. 120).

Classes of bronchodilator:

The commonly used bronchodilators fall into three classes:
a) β2–sympathomimetic
b) methyl xanthine
c) anticholinergic

β2 *sympathomimetics* are now highly β2 selective and unless given parenterally have little or no cardiac side effects. They are best given by pressurised inhaler provided the patient is technically competent with the device. Rotahalers, Spacers and pear-tube adaptors enable some of the patients who cannot use a pressurised inhaler to benefit from inhaled therapy. When given as tablets: $β_2$ sympathomimetics are not as effective as per inhaler and frequently cause tremor.

Nebuliser solutions are available and are especially useful in severe airways obstruction both in hospital and at home. In status asthmaticus parenteral formulations can be used but may aggravate hypoxaemia unless oxygen is also given. Intravenously they also cause tremor and tacycardia and should not be used together with intravenous aminophylline.

Methyl xanthines are used in the form of theophylline or aminophylline tablets in moderately severe airways obstruction. In status asthmaticus aminophylline is given intravenously by slow bolus injections or by constant infusion for 24–48 hours. Nausea, tremor, insomnia and tacycardia occur in 30–40% of those given methyl xanthines and limit their usefulness in day to day management. Slow-realease preparations are available, with the convenience of twice daily dosage and with less peak to trough variation in plasma levels. Suppositories give unpredictable plasma levels.

Anticholinergic therapy with I.M. atropine is effective but often causes unacceptable side-effects. For routine use ipratropium bro-

Table 7 Different forms of bronchodilator

	Preparation	Adult dose	Remarks
Pressurised inhaler	Salbutamol†	2 puffs 4 hourly p.r.n.	Can all be used more frequently
	Terbutaline*	2 puffs 6 hourly p.r.n.	
	Rimiterol	2 puffs 2 hourly p.r.n.	Seek medical advice
	Fenoterol	2 puffs 8 hourly p.r.n.	if no relief.
	Ipratropium bromide	2 puffs 6 hourly p.r.n.	Slower onset
Tablet	Salbutamol	2–4 mg 6 hrly	Tremor
	Terbutaline	2.5–5 mg 8 hrly	can occur
	Aminophylline	Variable	See B.N.F. or
	Theophylline	Variable	manufacturers' data sheets
Intravenous	Salbutamol	3–20 µg/min	Tacycardia
Subcutaneous	Terbutaline	250–500 µg 6 hourly	and tremor
or intravenous		1.5–5 µg/min	can occur
Intravenous	Aminophylline	5 mg/kg over 20 min then 1 mg/kg/hr; or 250–500 mg i.v. bolus slowly, 6 hourly.	Tacycardia, tremor and nausea can occur
Nebuliser solution	Salbutamol	5 mg in 4 ml	Use 8 l/m
	Terbutaline	5 mg in 4 ml	flow rate
	Ipratropium bromide	0.5 mg in 4 ml	

† Rotahaler available
* Spacer and Pear-tube adaptor available

mide by pressurised inhaler or nebuliser solution is effective and does not cause unpleasant atropinic symptoms.

Failure of symptoms to respond to increased use of bronchodilators is an indication that the patient should seek medical advice urgently. Methyl xanthines and sympathomimetics usually act additively, and can be synergistic towards both wanted and unwanted effects. Inhaled β2 sympathomimetic is often given together with systemic methyl xanthine but they should not be given systemically together. Ipratropium bromide acts additively with inhaled β2 sympathomimetic.

CORTICOSTEROID THERAPY

Indications for treatment.

Corticosteroids produce dramatic relief of airways obstruction in asthma, probably by reducing the local hypersenitivity reaction and the bronchial oedema. An acute asthma attack which necessitates admission to hospital is a life threatening condition and should always be treated with corticosteroids. Long term treatment with corticosteroids is indicated in chronic asthma not adequately controlled by regular bronchodilators and/or cromoglycate provided serial measurements of FEV_1 or PEFR show that corticosteroids produce significant improvement in ventilatory function (p. 120). Because of the numerous side effects, long term systemic treatment should never be prescribed casually. Corticosteroids are not effective in chronic bronchitis and emphysema.

Corticosteroids may prevent progressive pulmonary fibrosis in sarcoidosis and fibrosing alveolitis and long term treatment should be monitored with serial pulmonary function tests. Corticosteroids are also used in severe allergic alveolitis and together with anti-tuberculosis drugs in certain forms of tuberculosis.

Methods of adminstration.

In acute severe asthma (status asthmaticus) large doses of intravenous hydrocortisone and oral prednisolone are used initially. In long term treatment the inhaled corticosteroids, beclomethasone dipropionate and betamethasone valerate, are used in conjunction with bronchodilator and/or cromoglycate therapy. If control of symptoms is still not satisfactory prednisolone tablets are added, the maintenance doses being kept as low as is consistent with acceptable control (usually 5–10 mg. daily). Some patients will require just short, high-dose courses of prednisolone (20–30 mg daily for 3–5 days) whilst others will require regular therapy, with occasional short, high-dose boosts.

Inhaled corticosteroids in doses up to 1000 µg daily are free of systemic unwanted effects. Symptomatic oro-pharyngeal candidiasis occurs in 5–10% of patients but will usually respond to anti-fungal lozenges. Long-term systemic corticosteroids can cause osteoporosis with easy fracture, oedema, hypertension, hyperglycaemia, cataract and the classical Cushingoid facies. In children requiring long-term systemic corticosteroids corticotrophin injections (ACTH) are frequently used as this causes less retardation of growth than oral corticosteroids.

Patients on long term corticosteroids should carry a card giving this information in case they have a serious accident or require emergency surgery. It is the doctor's responsibility to inform the anaesthetist when one of his patients on corticosteroids is going for surgery. The dose of corticosteroids should be increased when patients on long term treatment are subjected to stressful situations. Long-term corticosteroids should never be stopped abruptly because this may cause severe exacerbation of symptoms. The dose should be reduced gradually over a period of months.

SODIUM CROMOGLYCATE (INTAL)

This compound inhibits mediator release from mast cells and is useful as a prophylactic in extrinsic asthma. To be effective it must be taken regularly, the majority of patients requiring four times daily dosage. It is inhaled as a dry powder (20 mg cromoglycate) from a punctured capsule via a Spinhaler. Occasionally patients find the powder irritant locally, a problem that can be solved by using inhaled bronchodilator before cromoglycate. Like sympathomimetic inhalers, cromoglycate used 10–15 minutes before exercise will usually block exercise induced asthma.

SEDATIVES AND ANALGESICES

Extreme caution must be used in giving sedatives and analgesics to patients with respiratory disease because of the risk of causing respiratory depression. Patients with asthma, chronic bronchitis and other chronic pulmonary diseases are particularly susceptible to barbiturates, tranquillizers and opiates and even trivial doses may be fatal. Barbiturates and opiates should never be given to patients with status asthmaticus or severe chronic bronchitis and emphysema. It must be remembered that restlessness and anxiety are common signs of hypoxaemia and must not be misinterpreted as psychological symptoms requiring treatment with sedatives.

Pethidine may be necessary to relieve pleuritic pain in pneumonia but must be used judiciously. Opiates should be given frequently and in adequate doses to relieve pain in patients with proven malignancy.

PHYSIOTHERAPY

The physiotherapist makes an important contribution to the management of patients with respiratory disease. Her help is invaluable in maintaining the patient's airway in respiratory failure. Assisted coughing is essential in exacerbations of chronic bronchitis and emphysema, bronchopneumonia and in clearing the viscid plugs of mucus in asthma attacks. Postural drainage is of value in bronchiectasis while pre- and post-operative physiotherapy will often prevent pulmonary complications after surgery.

THE PATIENT AS A PERSON

Illness frequently causes social and financial problems. The good doctor enquires about his patient's domestic responsibilities, financial commitments and work prospects. Tuberculosis, chronic bronchitis and emphysema and chronic asthma often give rise to social problems because of prolonged hospitalization. Bronchial carcinoma is accompanied by special problems because the expectation of life is short and frequently the patient has a young family. The medical social worker has the knowledge, skill and resources to help with these problems, and in enlightened centres the doctor meets her regularly to discuss patients' problems.

Illness always causes anxiety. It is the doctor's privilege to allay anxiety with explanation and kindness.

FURTHER READING

British Thoracic & Tuberculosis Association 1975 Inhaled corticosteroids compared with oral prednisone in patients staring long-term corticosteroid therapy for asthma. Lancet ii: 469
British Thoracic & Tuberculosis Association 1976 A controlled trial of inhaled corticosteroids in patients receiving prednisone tablets for asthma. British Journal of cases of the Dis. Chest 70:95
Cotes J E 1979 Lung function. 4th edn. Blackwell, Oxford
Crofton J Douglas A 1981 Respiratory diseases. 3rd edn. Blackwell, Oxford
Lancet 1981 Acute oxygen therapy. Lancet i:980
Patterson J N, Shenfield GM 1974 Bronchodilators Parts I and II. British Thoracic and Tuberculosis Association Review (suppl. to Tubercle) 4, 25:61.
Scottish Home and Health Department: Scottish Health Services Council. Report of a Sub-Committee of the Standing Medical Advisory Committee 1969 Uses and dangers of oxygen therapy. H M S O, Edinburgh

7

Upper respiratory tract infections and acute bronchitis

CLASSIFICATION OF ACUTE RESPIRATORY INFECTIONS

The terminology of acute respiratory infections is confusing because of the conflicting names given to different syndromes. An anatomical classification is unsatisfactory because many infections are not confined to a single site in the respiratory tract. An aetiological classification is impractical because over 100 different viruses and numerous types of bacteria cause respiratory infections and in many cases it is difficult to determine the aetiological agent. In addition, most organisms do not give rise to illnesses with distinctive clinical features. The classification adopted by the Medical Research Council is simple and practical (Table 8).

The MRC classification accounts for the majority of acute respiratory infections but omits conditions such as laryngitis and tracheitis which may occur alone but usually form part of one of the named syndromes. The term 'feverish cold' is used to describe an illness which is more incapacitating than the common cold and causes systemic upset or fever; sore throat covers both tonsillitis and pharyngitis.

The main acute lower respiratory tract infections in adults are acute bronchitis (p. 71) and pneumonia (p. 74). Attacks of acute bronchitis are common in adults with chronic bronchitis and are called exacerbations of chronic bronchitis (p. 129). 'Croup' is the name given to laryngotracheobronchitis of infancy and early childhood. The term 'bronchiolitis' is confined to acute bronchiolar infection in infants and is usually due to respiratory syncytial (RS) virus.

Table 8 Classification of acute respiratory infections

Upper respiratory infections	Lower respiratory infections
Common cold	Acute bronchitis
Feverish cold	Pneumonia
Sore throat	Croup (infants, young children)
Influenza	Bronchiolitis (infants)

UPPER RESPIRATORY TRACT INFECTIONS

Aetiology

Viruses are the predominant cause of acute upper respiratory tract infections. Table 9 shows a classification of the respiratory viruses and Table 10 outlines the principal organisms associated with the different types of infection. Each virus may cause a number of different clinical syndromes, and in turn each syndrome may be caused by a number of different viruses. The viruses responsible for a particular syndrome vary from year to year and from community to community. Viruses are recovered from only a small proportion of patients with presumed viral infections because of the technical difficulties of virus isolation.

Table 9 Classification of the respiratory viruses

Viruses	Serotypes
Influenza	A, B, C,
Parainfluenza	1, 2, 3, 4,
Respiratory syncytial (RS) virus	1
Rhinovirus	90+
Coxsackie	A: 1 to 24
	B: 1 to 6
Echo	30+
Adenovirus	30+

Table 10 Principal aetiological agents associated with acute upper respiratory tract infections

Infection	Principal agent
Common cold	Rhinovirus
	Parainfluenza
	RS virus
	Echo 28
	Coxsackie A21
Feverish cold	Adenovirus
	Rhinovirus
	Influenza
Sore throat	Adenovirus
	β haemolytic streptococci
Influenza	Influenza A, B, C

Laboratory diagnosis of viral infection

Virus isolation. Virus isolation may be attempted from nasopharyngeal washings, throat swabs and sputum. Sputum is collected in a sterile container but nasopharyngeal washings and throat swabs are collected in a suitable transport medium. Since respiratory viruses are very labile, specimens are stored at 4°C. The freezing compartment of a household refridgerator is suitable for overnight storage. If it is necessary to keep specimens for more than 48 hours they are stored at −70°C. With the advent of specific antiviral therapy, methods of virus isolation will assume greater clinical importance.

Serology. Paired specimens of sera are routinely tested. A fourfold rise in antibody titre between the first specimen, taken at the onset of the illness, and the second specimen, taken 2 to 3 weeks later, is diagnostic of current infection. Serological testing for rhinoviruses and echo viruses is not carried out routinely because of the numerous serotypes.

Immunity in viral infections

Interferon is produced by the infected host cells and plays an important role in preventing the spread of infection particularly in non-immune persons. Interferon interferes with the synthesis of viruses and a rise in serum interferon level precedes the rise in level of circulating antibody. Viral infections stimulate production of circulating IgG antibody and locally produced IgA antibody. Both are responsible for preventing reinfection but IgA is of major importance. IgA is manufactured by the plasma cells of the respiratory mucosa and is the predominant immunoglobulin in respiratory secretions.

Recurrent viral infections are common and may be explained by several different mechanisms. Reinfections with the same serotype may occur when the level of existing secretory antibody against the serotype has fallen. Reinfection may also occur as a result of infection with a serotype which has not been encountered previously. This serotype will be relatively insusceptible to antibodies produced by previous infections with other serotypes. There are over 90 different serotypes of rhinovirus and this partly explains why the common cold is common! Repeated attacks of influenza are the result of changes in the antigenic structures of the virus resulting in a new strain against which the individual is not protected by existing antibodies.

All these factors are of importance in the preparation of antiviral vaccines. Inactivated virus vaccines stimulate production of IgG but not IgA and confer less immunity than live attenuated vaccines which produce local secretory IgA antibody as well as IgG antibody. Research is continuing for effective vaccines; an effective common cold vaccine must confer immunity against the numerous serotypes of rhinovirus while an influenza vaccine must be effective against the current antigenic variant.

Epidemiology

Upper respiratory tract infections are an important cause of illness in the community and are the reason why 50 per cent of all patients consult their family doctor. In Britain, each person suffers an average of three respiratory infections per year. Acute respiratory infections are the major cause of absence from school and work and the economic effects of this are staggering. The common cold and influenza are responsible for 85 per cent of all acute respiratory infections and morbidity is highest in children less than 5 years of age. Children are particularly susceptible to viral infections until they have developed protective antibodies, and they are often responsible for introducing infection into the home. Mortality rates are highest in the young and in the elderly.

The method of spread of acute respiratory infections is by inhalation of infected droplets discharged into the air during talking, coughing and sneezing. Infections are more common in the winter months and this is related to overcrowding and seasonal variations in the prevalence of certain viruses. Influenza, parainfluenza and RS virus are prevalent during the winter months and often cause short outbreaks of community infection. Coxsackie and Echo are prevalent during the summer months, while rhinoviruses are present throughout the year but are isolated more commonly during autumn.

The nature and severity of upper respiratory infections are determined by the infecting virus and its virulence, the age and immune status of the individual, the occurrence of secondary bacterial infection and the presence of pre-existing respiratory disease.

Influenza

The epidemic nature of influenza has been known for centuries.

Influenza A causes pandemics (world wide epidemics) and in 1918 was responsible for 20 million deaths. Pandemics occur at irregular intervals but epidemics of varying severity occur at intervals of 2 to 3 years. This periodicity is due to changes in antigenic structure which render the virus insusceptible to existing antibodies. An epidemic wanes after a high proportion of the population have had influenza. Minor antigenic changes are responsible for less widespread outbreaks of infection.

Three antigens of the influenza virus are known to be important. The ribonucleoprotein is an internal antigen and determines the virus type, i.e. types A, B and C. Influenza A virus is subtyped by identifying the two surface antigens, haemagglutinin and neuraminidase. The haemagglutinin is the main antigen responsible for establishing infection and for provoking the production of neutralizing antibodies. New strains of influenza A virus are named according to the place and date of isolation, and their haemagglutinin and neuraminidase antigenic structure, e.g. influenza A/Singapore/1/57 (H_2 N_2) and A/Hong Kong/1/68 (H_3 N_2). This indicates that the haemagglutinin of A/Hong Kong/68 is different from that of the preceding strain but the neuraminidase is the same.

World Health Organization Influenza Centres in different countries maintain a constant vigilance for new strains of influenza A. When a new strain appears they characterize its antigenic structure and follow its path of spread.

Influenza B may also cause epidemics but these are less widespread than influenza A epidemics. Influenza C causes only sporadic infection.

Pathology and functional abnormality

The principal pathological changes are oedema, hyperaemia and hypersecretion of the mucosa of the upper respiratory tract. Influenza also involves the trachea and bronchi and causes desquamation of the mucosa, ciliary damage and increased secretions, which predispose to secondary bacterial infection and may result in pneumonia. Occasionally viruses cause pneumonia uncomplicated by bacterial infection. Such cases show desquamation of the alveolar cells, a hyaline membrane lining the alveoli, and thrombosis, necrosis and haemorrhage of the pulmonary capillaries.

The pathological changes produce local and general effects. The inflammation of the respiratory mucosa may cause difficulty in breathing and troublesome secretions while systemic symptoms result from absorption of toxic products and occasionally from viraemia.

Clinical features

Common cold (coryza)

After an incubation period of 2 to 3 days the patient notices dryness and irritation of the throat, nasal congestion, sneezing and profuse watery nasal discharge. The eyes become inflamed and the voice husky. The patient feels lethargic and develops a cough productive of mucoid sputum. Severe constitutional symptoms and fever are uncommon. The acute symptoms subside within a few days but the nasal discharge and cough may persist for a week or more. Acute sinusitis and otitis media may complicate the common cold.

The differential diagnosis includes *allergic rhinitis* in which the sudden onset of sneezing and nasal discharge can often be attributed to contact with an allergen such as pollen or house dust. The *acute exanthemata* often begin with symptoms suggestive of a cold, but the diagnosis becomes obvious when the rash appears.

Feverish cold

The feverish cold is similar to the common cold but causes fever and systemic symptoms. It is a more severe and prolonged illness than the common cold but is less severe than influenza.

Sore throat

This syndrome comprises marked sore throat, malaise and fever. The pharynx and tonsils are inflamed and may be covered with exudate. In severe cases the upper cervical lymph nodes are painful and enlarged. Viral and streptococcal sore throat cannot be distinguished clinically and it is advisable to take a throat swab for bacterial culture because sometimes β haemolytic streptococci are responsible. Adenoviruses often cause outbreaks of sore throat in service personnel.

Influenza

The symptoms of influenza begin suddenly after an incubation period of about 48 hours. Symptoms are predominantly systemic in nature and include fever, shivering, malaise, aching limbs, headache, backache and anorexia. Nasal symptoms, sore throat and dry cough are common. The physical signs include watering and injection of the eyes and redness of the pharynx. Chest signs are uncommon. Delirium and atrial fibrillation occasionally develop during the acute stage of the illness. The fever and constitutional symptoms subside after several days, but there is often persistent productive cough and sometimes prolonged lassitude and depression.

Pneumonia is the most serious complication and occurs synchronously with influenza or may follow it. Pneumonia complicating influenza is sometimes a fulminating illness with respiratory and peripheral circulatory failure. It is usually due to *Staph. aureus* or *Str. pneumoniae* but may be a primary influenza virus pneumonia. Pneumonia is commonest in those with pre-existing chest and cardiac disease, but during influenza epidemics fulminating pneumonia is not uncommon in healthy young people. Other complications include bronchitis, and rarely pericarditis, myocarditis and encephalitis. Another rare complication is disseminated intravascular coagulation which causes generalized bleeding, anaemia, thrombocytopenia and defibrination.

Influenza-like illness is common and may be caused by adenoviruses, parainfluenza, coxsackie and *M. pneumoniae*. The clinical features resemble influenza and the precise aetiology can only be determined by laboratory investigations.

Treatment

There is no specific therapy for upper respiratory tract infections since the majority are caused by viruses. If the patient is febrile or feels ill he should rest. Paracetamol or soluble aspirin gives symptomatic relief and a mild hypnotic induces a restful sleep. Adequate fluids are essential, especially in children and old people who are liable to become dehydrated.

Antibiotics are not indicated in most cases. Penicillin is given if β haemolytic streptococci are isolated from patients with sore throat or if pneumonia develops as a complication. It is combined with flucloxacillin, cloxacillin or methicillin in suspected or proven staphylococcal pneumonia (p. 87). Prophylactic tetracycline, 250 mg 6 hourly, is often given to patients with chronic chest disease or cardiac failure when they develop an upper respiratory infection, because of the increased risk of bronchitis and pneumonia.

Prognosis and prevention

Upper respiratory tract infections are self limiting and usually the prognosis is good. Pneumonia complicating influenza has a 20 per cent mortality rate. Influenza vaccines are not sufficiently effective to justify nation wide immunization but some provide 60 per cent protection and it is advisable to vaccinate pregnant women and patients with chronic lung and cardiac disease.

Acute bronchitis

Acute bronchitis may be a primary infection of the respiratory tract but more commonly it develops as a complication of an upper respiratory tract infection or as an exacerbation of acute infection in chronic bronchitis and emphysema (p. 129). The usual causal organisms are *H. influenzae and Strep. pneumoniae.*

Cough, mucopurulent sputum and wheeze are the common symptoms. Fever is not a constant feature and dyspnoea is not severe unless there is pre-existing pulmonary or heart disease. Rhonchi are usually present.

Acute bronchitis does not cause radiographic abnormalities and often there is no leucocytosis.

Ampicillin, 250 mg 8 hourly, is the antibiotic of choice and is usually given for 1 week. Steam inhalations provide symptomatic relief and assist expectoration. Acute bronchitis is usually a mild illness without complications. The differentiation between bronchitis and asthma is discussed on page 121.

Mycoplasmal infections

Mycoplasmal infections are common in domestic animals and poultry but *M. pneumoniae* is the only species known to cause disease in man. *M. pneumoniae* is mainly responsible for upper respiratory tract infections, although in about 5 per cent of infected persons it causes pneumonia. Infection is acquired by inhalation and occurs predominantly in children and young adults. Close contact favours spread of infection, and outbreaks occur among families and service personnel.

The clinical features of mycoplasmal infection are not sufficiently distinctive to allow a clinical diagnosis, although in some patients with mycoplasmal pneumonia the symptoms are predominantly systemic rather than respiratory.

M. pneumoniae may persist in the respiratory tract for several months after the onset of the illness and this may explain why persistent cough is common. Mycoplasmal infections are not usually serious but they may be accompanied by otitis media, haemolytic anaemia, the Stevens-Johnson syndrome and skin rashes. Demonstration of a fourfold rise in complement fixing antibodies is the routine method of diagnosis. Cold agglutinins develop in 50 per cent of cases.

M. pneumoniae is sensitive to tetracycline and erythromycin and treatment shortens the duration of the illness. Tetracycline, 500 mg 6 hourly, is given in suspected or proven infections.

Pleurodynia (Bornholm disease)

This disease is named after the Island of Bornholm in the Baltic Sea where early studies were carried out. Pleurodynia is caused by coxsackie B viruses and commonly occurs in small epidemics. Pleurodynia causes sudden pleuritic pain, fever, cough and headache. The pain is often localized to the region of the diaphragmatic attachment and may be mainly epigastric. Intercostal tenderness and hyperaesthesia are common at the site of the pain and a pleural rub may be present.

The diagnosis is confirmed by isolation of coxsackie B virus from throat washings or stools and by demonstration of a fourfold rise in antibodies. The illness is self limiting and treatment is symptomatic. Other diseases caused by coxsackie B viruses include aseptic meningitis, pericarditis, orchitis, and, in the infant, myocarditis.

FURTHER READING

British Medical Journal 1965 Report of the Medical Research Council Working Party. A collaborative study of the aetiology of acute respiratory infections in Britain 1961–64. 2: 319
Crofton J, Douglas A 1981 Respiratory diseases, 3rd Edn. Blackwell Scientific Publications, Oxford
Stuart-Harris C H 1976 Influenza: the virus and the disease. Wright PSG, London
Tyrrell D A J 1965 Common colds and related diseases. Arnold, London

8

Pneumonia

DEFINITION

Pneumonia is defined as inflammation of the lung which is characterized by exudation into the alveoli.

CLASSIFICATION

Pneumonia may be classified on an anatomical basis into *lobular pneumonia*, *lobar pneumonia*, or *segmental pneumonia*. The frequency of the different types is lobular 70 per cent, lobar 20 per cent and segmental 10 per cent. *Bronchopneumonia* is the term given to bilateral lobular pneumonia. Pneumonia may also be classified on an aetiological basis. However, the same causal agents do not cause pneumonia of specific anatomical distribution. Therefore both classifications are used to describe pneumonia, e.g. pneumococcal lobar pneumonia, pneumococcal bronchopneumonia.

The term 'pneumonitis' is synonymous with pneumonia and its use is unnecessary. 'Aspiration pneumonia' is a term applied to pneumonia presumed to be due to inhalation of foreign material, infected secretions, or gastro-intestinal contents. The name 'primary atypical pneumonia' was originally applied to pneumonias other than those caused by any known micro-organisms. This term, implying knowledge of an ideal and perfect pneumonia existing as it were in some platonic heaven, is not only meaningless, but confusing. 'I was once delighted to hear an incautious person refer to an atypical atypical pneumonia' (Scadding, 1948).

EPIDEMIOLOGY

Pneumonia is a common disease and approximately 1 per cent of the population suffer an attack each year. It affects all age groups and among adults about 50 per cent of cases occur under the age of 50.

Pneumonia is commonest in the winter and spring due to factors such as sudden falls in temperature, the seasonal prevalence of certain respiratory viruses and overcrowding. Overcrowding favours transmission of bacteria and viruses and is partly responsible for the higher incidence of pneumonia in the lower socio-economic groups. Alcoholism, cigarette smoking and atmospheric pollution are also associated with increased attack rates from pneumonia.

The mortality rate from pneumonia is 5 to 10 per cent. Death is commonest in the very young and the elderly. The infant and the young child are particularly susceptible because of poorly developed immune responses and relatively narrow airways which are easily occluded by secretions. In the aged, pneumonia is often the terminal event in those already handicapped by chronic disease.

PREDISPOSING CONDITIONS

Interference with the defence mechanisms of the respiratory tract may lead to inhalation of foreign material and accumulation of bronchial secretions, providing conditions which predispose to the development of pneumonia.

Inhalation of foreign material
This may occur whenever the level of consciousness is impaired and the cough reflex depressed, e.g. anaesthesia, acute alcoholism, drug overdose, neurological disorders. Inefficient expectoration and retention of bronchial secretions may give rise to pneumonia after surgery and chest trauma. Regurgitation and inhalation of food sometimes complicate oesophageal stricture and achalasia. Inhalation of small objects such as peanuts and stones may cause pneumonia in children.

Pre-existing respiratory disease
Viral infections of the upper or lower respiratory tract, particularly influenza, damage the respiratory epithelium and predispose to bacterial pneumonia. Chronic bronchitis and bronchiectasis are often complicated by pneumonia because of the inadequate drainage of bronchial secretions and the presence of intrabronchial pathogens. Pneumonia is sometimes the first manifestation of bronchial carcinoma and results from infection of retained secretions secondary to bronchial obstruction by tumour. Dental caries and chronic sinusitis also favour the development of pneumonia. Cystic fibrosis is characterized by production of abnormal mucus, and recurrent pneumonia is common. The mucus contains *p-hydroxy-phenylacetic acid*

which enhances the growth of *Staph. aureus* and possibly increases susceptibility to staphylococcal pneumonia.

Immunological disorders

Leukaemia, lymphoma, multiple myeloma and hypogammaglobulinaemia predispose to pneumonia; occasionally pneumonia is the first manifestation of these diseases. Patients receiving immunosupressive drugs are at greater risk of pneumonia.

AETIOLOGY

The majority of pneumonias are the result of infection. Many different types of organisms are capable of causing pneumonia, but bacteria are the commonest aetiological agents.

Bacterial pneumonias

Str. pneumoniae is responsible for 70–80 per cent of all pneumonias. The pneumococcus disappears rapidly from the sputum once antibiotics are started and it may not be isolated from patients admitted to hospital because they have often had antibiotics before admission. The pneumococcus has a well defined polysaccharide capsule which is type specific and is almost indigestible by phagocytes. There are more than 30 different types of pneumococci and the lower numbered types, 1 to 10, are of greater pathogenicity and more commonly cause pneumonia than the higher types. The type 3 pneumococcus is the most virulent. Pneumococci, usually the higher types, are isolated from the nasopharynx in 40 per cent of healthy people.

Staph. aureus causes 5 per cent of all pneumonias but the incidence often rises sharply during influenza epidemics. Staphylococcal pneumonia is often a severe illness which may be fulminating when it complicates influenza. The severity of the illness may be aggravated by the fact that the staphylococcus is frequently resistant to penicillin and is sometimes resistant to flucloxacillin and methicillin.

M. tuberculosis usually causes chronic inflammation of the lung characterized by fibrosis and cavitation, which by definition is not strictly classified as pneumonia. However, it is often initially difficult to differentiate from pneumonia, and for this reason it is justifiable to consider tuberculosis in the aetiology of pneumonia.

K. pneumoniae is responsible for about 1 per cent of all pneumonias. It causes pneumonia in alcoholics or elderly debilitated people and may give rise to abscesses in the upper lobes.

H. influenza causes bronchopneumonia in patients with chronic bronchitis and emphysema, especially the elderly. *E. coli, Proteus* and *Pseudomonas* rarely cause pneumonia. They frequently appear in the sputum of patients with pneumonia during antibiotic treatment. This is due to colonization of the ecological vacuum which remains after the primary pathogen has been eliminated. In this situation it is most unlikely that Gram negative bacteria play a pathogenic role, but they may be aetiologically significant if they are isolated repeatedly in heavy growth. Gram negative bacteria are occasionally responsible for pneumonia in patients with immunological disorders.

Pneumonia is sometimes a manifestation of specific bacterial diseases such as *pertussis, typhoid* and *brucellosis*.

Viral pneumonias

Many different viruses have been identified in association with pneumonia, e.g. *influenza, parainfluenza, adenovirus, respiratory syncytial virus*. Their role as primary causal agents is difficult to determine. Serological evidence of viral infection, usually influenza, is detected in about 15 per cent of patients admitted to hospital with pneumonia, but often pneumococci or staphylococci are isolated from these cases, and in the majority the pneumonia is due to secondary bacterial infection. Accordingly it is not strictly correct to classify these cases as viral pneumonia. Viruses are more likely to be the sole causal agents of pneumonia during epidemics of influenza or of adenoviral infection in service personnel. It is doubtful if respiratory syncytial virus or parainfluenza viruses are ever primary causal agents in adults.

Pneumonia may complicate systemic viral diseases like *varicella* and *measles*. Pneumonia is a complication of varicella in 30 per cent of cases and is usually caused by the virus itself, while pneumonia complicating measles is due to secondary bacterial infection.

Psittacosis

Psittacosis is caused by *C. psittaci* which shares some of the characteristics of rickettsiae and viruses. Psittacosis is primarily a disease of birds and is so named because it was first recognized in parrots which belong to the family *Psittacidae*. It has since been found in most types of birds. Human infection sometimes occurs in those who keep buderigars, pigeons and poultry, and is caused by inhalation of dust from the excreta of infected birds.

Mycoplasmal pneumonia

In 1944 Eaton identified a filterable agent from patients with 'atypical pneumonia'. Nearly 20 years passed before Eaton's agent was shown to be *M. pneumoniae*. This is the only species of mycoplasma known to cause respiratory disease in man and in most cases the infection is confined to the bronchial tree and pneumonia does not develop. Infection with *M. pneumoniae* can be demonstrated in about 15 per cent of patients admitted to hospital with pneumonia. Most mycoplasmal infections occur in late childhood or early adult life and close personal contact and a large susceptible population favour spread of infection. Outbreaks of mycoplasmal pneumonia, uncomplicated by bacterial infection, occur in service personnel and university students. Similar outbreaks have also been reported in families.

Q Fever
R. burneti causes Q fever which was first recognized as a new disease by Derrick in 1937, when he investigated an outbreak of febrile illness among workers in a Brisbane abattoir. Derrick called this disease Q fever. The Q was an abbreviation for 'query', signifying unknown facts about the disease, and did not refer to Queensland, the State in which it was first recognized. Q fever is a worldwide disease and predominantly affects cattle and sheep. Human infection is acquired by inhalation of rickettsiae from infected animals and occurs mainly in abattoir workers and farmers. Q fever causes a febrile illness characterized by headache, anorexia, myalgia and hepatosplenomegaly. Respiratory signs and symptoms occur in about 40 per cent of cases but the incidence of pneumonia is variable.

Legionnaire's disease
Legionella pneumophila, a Gram negative coccobacillus, caused an outbreak of pneumonia at a convention of Legionnaires in Philadelphia in 1976. The organism has been repeatedly isolated from water samples from air-conditioning systems or showers, which may account for its predilection for hotel and hospital populations. The diagnosis should be considered in any severe pneumonia with mucoid sputum especially if abdominal pain, diarrhoea and confusion are prominent features and the recent environmental history is suggestive.

Fungal pneumonias
Fungi cause a variety of reactions in the lung, including pneumonia. Fungal pneumonias are rare although *C. albicans* and *A. fumigatus* are occasionally responsible for pneumonia in patients with immunological disorders. These fungi are common saprophytes in the

environment and are sometimes isolated from sputum, particularly in patients on antibiotics. Usually this finding is not aetiologically significant.

Pneumonia in immunocompromised patients

In addition to an increased risk of infection by the common pathogens, these patients may develop pneumonia caused by *Pneumocystis carinii*, Cytomegalovirus and fungi (see above). Anaerobes can infect such patients, as well as causing pneumonia in other patients debilitated after abdominal surgery or who may have aspirated for any other reason.

PATHOGENESIS, PATHOLOGY AND FUNCTIONAL ABNORMALITY

Pneumonia usually results from inhalation of organisms but sometimes infection reaches the lung through the blood stream. Staphylococcal pneumonia often follows septicaemia secondary to staphylococcal skin infection. Bacteraemia occurs in 15 per cent of all pneumonias.

In lobular pneumonia there are scattered areas of inflammation in the bronchioles and alveoli which are filled with inflammatory exudate. In lobar pneumonia, outpouring of oedema fluid into the alveoli at the site of the initial infection facilitates spread of bacteria throughout the lobe. The alveoli become filled with red cells, fibrin and polymorphonuclear leucocytes. The lobe becomes congested and airless. Resolution occurs as the neutrophils engulf bacteria and are then ingested by macrophages. The inflammatory exudate is gradually absorbed and residual fibrosis is rare. Pneumonia frequently involves the pleura, causing fibrinous pleurisy, although pleural effusion and empyema are uncommon. Necrosis of lung tissue may give rise to lung abscess, but this is unusual except in staphylococcal and klebsiella pneumonias.

The physiological changes in pneumonia are mainly due to the intra-alveolar exudate. In extensive pneumonia blood is shunted through the affected lung without being adequately oxygenated and the P_aO_2 falls. Increased ventilation of normal lung keeps the P_aCO_2 normal, or it may even be reduced. However, hyperventilation cannot compensate for the hypoxaemia, because blood leaving normal lung tissue is already almost fully oxygenated. Patients with chronic bronchitis may be unable to hyperventilate sufficiently to prevent a rise in P_aCO_2, while in normal persons hypercapnia develops if excessive secretions interfere with ventilation. Pneumonia increases the stiffness of the lung so that the compliance is reduced and the work of breathing is increased; to compensate the respiratory rate rises.

These pathological and functional changes account for the symptoms of pneumonia: cough, purulent sputum, breathlessness, fever and malaise. The intra-alveolar exudate gives rise to crepitations. In lobar pneumonia the breath sounds are bronchial in quality because the consolidated lobe acts as a good conducting medium for the sounds produced by the movement of air through the trachea and large bronchi.

CLINICAL FEATURES

It has been customary to consider the clinical features of pneumonia according to the anatomical type and the aetiological agent. Many patients are now treated early in their illness with antibiotics which modify the symptoms and signs. Often the clinical picture is not sufficiently distinctive to allow an accurate anatomical or aetiological diagnosis. In practice, it is more important to recognize the clinical features common to all pneumonias.

Onset. The onset is characteristically sudden with rigors or pleuritic pain in pneumococcal lobar pneumonia. In other types of pneumonia the onset is often insidious and symptoms arise over a few days. Frequently there is a history of a recent upper respiratory tract infection.

Cough and sputum. Initially the cough is dry but after a few days it becomes productive of purulent sputum. Sometimes the sputum is streaked with blood, but profuse haemoptysis is uncommon.

Breathlessness. This is common if the pneumonia is extensive or if the patient's respiratory function is poor.

Pleuritic pain. Sometimes the patient complains of chest pain, which is sharp in quality and is aggravated by coughing or by taking a deep breath. The pain may be referred to the shoulder or upper abdomen.

Fever, anorexia and malaise. Systemic symptoms are common although fever may be slight or absent in elderly patients.

Mental confusion. Severe pneumonia may cause mental confusion due to hypoxaemia, hypercapnia or hypotension.

Physical examination. The patient is often dyspnoeic and uses the accessory muscles of respiration. The respiratory rate and depth are increased and the pulse is rapid. The patient appears flushed and may have central cyanosis.

On examination of the chest the commonest finding is the presence of coarse crepitations in one or both lower lobes. This is often the only abnormality in bronchopneumonia, although localized bronchial breathing may be heard if there is patchy bronchopneumonic consolidation. The classical signs of consolidation are not common and mainly occur in pneumococcal lobar pneumonia: the chest movement is reduced on the affected side, the percussion note is dull and the breath sounds are bronchial over the affected lobe (p. 43). Increased vocal fremitus and particularly increased vocal resonance with whispering pectoriloquy confirm the presence of lobar consolidation.

A pleural friction rub is often heard, particularly in patients with pleuritic pain.

The severity of the illness is variable and depends upon the extent of the pneumonia, the patient's respiratory function, the aetiological agent and whether bacteraemia is present. If the patient is desperately ill with mental confusion, central cyanosis and peripheral circulatory failure, it is important to suspect staphylococcal pneumonia. The likelihood of staphylococcal pneumonia is increased if there is a history of a 'flu-like illness or if the patient presents during an influenza epidemic. Pneumococcal bacteraemia also causes a severe illness. Sometimes there are few respiratory symptoms and no systemic upset, and the diagnosis is only made when a chest radiograph is taken because of minor symptoms.

Viral pneumonia may cause predominantly systemic symptoms with marked headache, malaise and muscle pain accompanied by irritating cough, mucoid sputum and few physical signs in the chest. However, it is often impossible to differentiate clinically between viral pneumonia and bacterial pneumonia. Similarly a clinical diagnosis of mycoplasmal pneumonia cannot be made with accuracy. One clue which suggests the possibility of viral or mycoplasmal infection is a history of a recent cold or 'flu-like illness, particularly if other members of the family have had a similar illness.

A clinical diagnosis of psittacosis, Q fever or Legionnaire's should be considered if there is relevant occupational or environmental exposure. These diseases are rarely identified from the symptoms and signs alone.

INVESTIGATIONS

Chest radiograph. A chest radiograph should always be taken to confirm the diagnosis and to help to exclude tuberculosis and bronchial carcinoma. Lobar pneumonia appears as a homogeneous opacity bounded by the fissures of the lung (Figs. 7, 8, 9). It does not

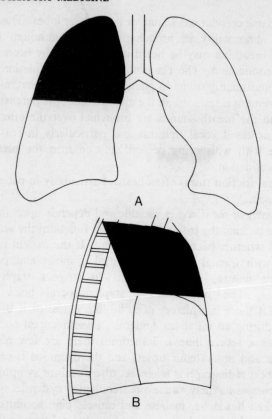

Fig. 7 Lobar pneumonia, right upper lobe. (a) PA view; (b) lateral view. The homogeneous opacity is limited on its inferior aspect by the horizontal fissure.

cause mediastinal displacement unless there is associated collapse. Segmental pneumonia also causes a localized homogeneous opacity, but its outline is less clearly defined. Patchy areas of non-homogeneous shadowing, in the mid or lower zones, are characteristic of lobular pneumonia or bronchopneumonia (Figs. 10, 11). Sometimes bronchopneumonia causes miliary mottling.

Sputum examination. Before starting antibiotic treatment sputum is collected for Gram stain and culture. If the patient is desperately ill the Gram film should be examined immediately, since demonstration of organisms resembling staphylococci influences the choice of antibiotic. It is important to appreciate that although bacteria may be isolated from sputum they may not be the causal agent. Gram negative bacteria are rarely significant unless repeatedly isolated in heavy growth.

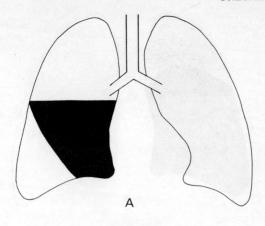

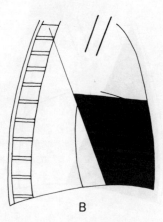

Fig. 8 Pneumonia, middle lobe. (a) PA view; (b) Lateral view. The homogeneous opacity is bounded by the horizontal and oblique fissures.

The sputum should also be examined for tubercle bacilli.

Blood culture. This should be carried out routinely since bacteria isolated from the blood are of more aetiological significance than bacteria isolated from sputum. A positive blood culture may subsequently affect antibiotic treatment.

Viral and mycoplasmal studies. Paired sera are examined for viral and mycoplasmal antibodies and if facilities are available sputum is cultured for these organisms. Psittacosis, Rickettsia and Legionella titres are also measured.

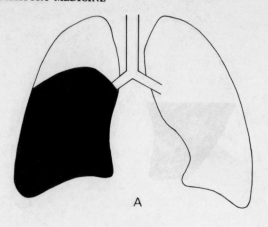

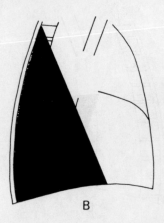

Fig. 9 Lobar pneumonia, right lower lobe. (a) PA view; (b) Lateral view. The homogeneous opacity occupies the mid and lower zones and is bounded anteriorly by the oblique fissure.

Peripheral blood. Commonly the white cell count rises to 12 000 to 16 000/m^3, but 20 per cent of patients do not develop leucocytosis and have a normal ESR. Leucopenia sometimes occurs in severe pneumonia.

Blood gas analysis. This is advisable, unless the patient is only mildly ill, because hypoxaemia is often more severe than is suspected clinically. Knowledge of the $P_{a}CO_2$ facilitates the correct choice of oxygen concentration and reduces the risk of causing carbon dioxide narcosis.

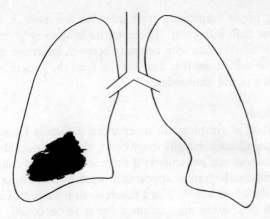

Fig. 10 Lobular pneumonia. The differential diagnosis of a localized ill-defined non homogeneous opacity includes pulmonary infarction, tuberculosis and bronchial carcinoma.

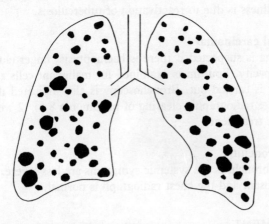

Fig. 11 Bilateral lobular pneumonia: bronchopneumonia. Diffuse nodular opacities. The differential diagnosis includes tuberculosis, metastatic carcinoma, pneumoconiosis and sarcoidosis.

DIFFERENTIAL DIAGNOSIS

Pulmonary infarction

Pleuritic pain, sudden breathlessness and haemoptysis are characteristic of pulmonary infarction but are present in only 50 per cent of patients, and often it is impossible to distinguish between infarction and peumonia. The legs should be examined carefully for evidence of deep vein thrombosis and attention paid to possible factors which may have predisposed to infarction. Purulent sputum and a preceding upper respiratory tract infection are more in favour of pneumonia than infarction. There are no laboratory investigations which will differentiate with certainty between infarction and pneumonia, and sometimes it is necessary to treat the patient with both anticoagulants and antibiotics.

Tuberculosis

The duration of symptoms in tuberculosis is usually longer than in pneumonia. Chronic cough, weight loss, night sweats and ill health favour tuberculosis, particularly if there is a history of contact. The characteristic radiographic appearance is patchy shadowing and cavitation in the upper zones. When tuberculosis is suspected additional specimens of sputum are examined for tubercle bacilli. A strong positive tuberculin test is in favour of tuberculosis but is not diagnostic. If a previous chest radiograph shows an apical abnormality consistent with an old tuberculous lesion it is more likely that the present illness is due to reactivation of tuberculosis.

Bronchial carcinomal

Carcinoma is suspected if there is haemoptysis, finger clubbing or a hilar opacity. Sputum is examined for malignant cells and bronchoscopy is carried out. Bronchoscopy is also indicated if there is incomplete radiographic clearing of pneumonia 8 to 12 weeks after antibiotic treatment.

Acute bronchitis

In acute bronchitis the systemic symptoms are less severe, pleuritic pain is absent and the chest radiograph is normal.

TREATMENT

Antibiotics

Penicillin or ampicillin are the antibiotics of choice because the majority of pneumonias are due to the pneumococcus which is virtually always sensitive to these drugs. Penicillin is given as I.M. benzyl penicillin, 1 mega unit bd; oral penicillin should not be used initially because it may not achieve adequate blood levels. Ampicillin 250 mg 6–hourly is often preferred to penicillin because it is equally effective and avoids the necessity of injections. Antibiotic treatment is continued for 1 to 2 weeks.

Tetracycline or erythromycin, 2 g daily, are given if the patient is allergic to penicillin or if mycoplasmal pneumonia, psittacosis, Q

fever or Legionnaire's are suspected. The antibiotic treatment of
staphylococcal pneumonia is discussed below.

When   K. pneumoniae is isolated, sensitivity tests are used as a
guide for the selection of the appropriate antibiotics. Metronidazole
is used for anaerobes.

Oxygen

35 per cent oxygen is administered when cyanosis is present but if
there is reason to suspect previous CO_2 retention, 24–28 per cent
oxygen is given by Ventimask.

General measures

The patient's airway must be kept clear by regular supervised coughing. Adequate fluids are given and the fluid intake recorded. Analgesics such as pethidine may be necessary to relieve pleuritic pain
but must be used with care to avoid respiratory depression.

Desperately ill patient

The treatment of the desperately ill patient differs from that of the
patient who is not very sick. Treatment is directed towards adequate
antibiotic cover and correction of respiratory failure and peripheral
circulatory failure.

It should be assumed that staphylococci are the causal agent,
especially if they are seen on the Gram stain or isolated from sputum.
Until the results of sensitivity tests are known it should be assumed
that the staphylococci are resistant to penicillin, and flucloxacillin
500 mg is given 4 to 6 hourly by injection. Flucloxacillin is more
effective when given in combination with benzyl penicillin, 1 mega
unit 6 hourly. Erythromycin, lincomycin or fusidic acid are given
if the patient is allergic to penicillin.

When the patient is desperately ill the possibility of klebsiella
pneumonia and tuberculosis must also be considered, and antibiotics
effective against these organisms are often given until the causal
agent is identified.

Course and prognosis

Usually the patient becomes afebrile and shows clinical improvement within 3 to 4 days of starting antibiotics. The degree of sputum
purulence is a good indication of progress, and in most cases the
sputum is mucoid within ten days. The radiographic abnormalities
start to clear by the second week of treatment, although the average
time taken to achieve maximum radiographic clearing is six weeks.

The mortality rate is 5 to 10 per cent. The main factors which influence prognosis are the age of the patient, the causal organism and the presence of bacteraemia. Bacteraemic pneumococcal pneumonia treated with antibiotics has a mortality of up to 20 per cent.

Delayed resolution

It is imperative that the patient is kept under observation until the radiograph is normal or has returned to its previous appearance. Comparison with previous radiographs will sometimes show that residual abnormalities have been present for some years and consequently are of little significance. If incomplete radiographic clearing cannot be attributed to previous pulmonary disease it is important to carry out sputum cytology and bronchoscopy to exclude bronchial carcinoma. These investigations should not be delayed if resolution is incomplete, and sometimes thoracotomy is necessary to determine the nature of a persistent abnormality. The sputum should always be examined for *M. tuberculosis* if pneumonia is slow to resolve.

Complications

Respiratory failure. Central cyanosis indicates respiratory failure but is not obvious until there is severe hypoxaemia. Hypercapnia may be present if chronic bronchitis or retained secretions prevent adequate ventilation. For these reasons blood gas analysis is advisable in all but the mildest cases. Ventilatory failure can often be prevented by regular assisted coughing and physiotherapy. Sometimes bronchoscopic aspiration or intubation are necessary if copious secretions obstruct the main airways. Tracheostomy and assisted ventilation are rarely required.

Peripheral circulatory failure. This serious complication is usually due to staphylococcal septicaemia or pneumococcal bacteraemia. It is treated with plasma expanders although care must be taken not to overload the circulation. Corticosteroids are usually given in large doses; hydrocortisone 1000 mg I.V. in the first 24 hours.

Lung abscess.

This is a complication in 2 per cent of patients. *Staph. aureus* is the usual causal agent, particularly in children with cystic fibrosis. *K. pneumoniae* may cause abscesses in the upper lobes. Persistent fever and purulent sputum are characteristic of lung abscess but may not occur if the abscess is small. The chest radiograph shows a circumscribed area of translucency with a fluid level in the region of the pneumonic shadowing. Further specimens of sputum should be examined for bacteria, tubercle bacilli and malignant cells. Persistence of a lung abscess is an indication for bronchoscopy to exclude bronchial carcinoma or foreign body. Treatment is discussed on page 96.

Pleural effusion. Effusion occurs in 5 per cent of patients and may cause persistent fever or recurrence of fever during convalescence. If there is more than a thin layer of fluid, pleural aspiration is carried out to prevent the development of empyema. Postpneumonic effusion is an exudate and the predominant cell type is the polymorph. When aspiration is necessary a pleural biopsy is taken, since this helps to exclude other causes of effusion. Recurrence after aspiration is uncommon in pneumonia and suggests the possibility of tumour, pulmonary infarction or tuberculosis.

Empyema. This occurs in less than 1 per cent of cases and causes persistent fever, cough and weight loss (p. 98).

Cardiac failure. Pneumonia may precipitate or aggravate cardiac failure in elderly patients.

Hypersensitivity to penicillin.
This develops in about 5 per cent of patients. The usual signs are rash and fever on the 7th to 10th days of treatment. Sometimes fever is the only manifestation. This may be misleading but can be detected by temporarily stopping penicillin and observing the effect on the temperature.

Deep vein thrombosis. Venous thrombosis may occur if immobilization is prolonged, and is another cause of fever during convalescence.

Causes of failure of treatment
Table 11 shows the causes of failure of pneumonia to respond to treatment. The commonest cause is incorrect diagnosis. Pulmonary infarction, tuberculosis and bronchial carcinoma are the conditions most likely to be confused with pneumonia. A careful review of the history and relevant investigations will usually establish the correct diagnosis.

If the patient fails to show clinical improvement or is still febrile after treatment for five days it is possible that the organism is resistant. *Staph. aureus* and *K. pneumoniae* are the causal agents most commonly insensitive to penicillin or ampicillin and can usually be isolated readily from fresh specimens of sputum. It is also worth considering the possibility of mycoplasmal pneumonia, psittacosis, Q fever or Legionnaire's.If history suggests that these organisms could be responsible tetracycline or erythromycin, 2 g daily, should be given. It is helpful to obtain the results of the complement fixation tests on the first specimen of serum; a high titre is suggestive of recent infection.

Delayed response to treatment may be due to complications such as lung abscess, pleural effusion or empyema.

Table 11 Causes of failure of pneumonia to respond to treatment

Incorrect diagnosis
  Pulmonary infarction
  Tuberculosis
  Bronchial carcinoma
Organisms resistant to penicillin
  Staph. aureus
  K. pneumoniae
  M. pneumoniae
  C. psittaci (psittacosis)
  R. burneti (Q fever)
  L. pneumophila (Legionnaire's)
Complications of pneumonia
  Lung abscess
  Pleural effusion
  Empyema

RECURRENT PNEUMONIA

When a patient has recurrent attacks of pneumonia an attempt must be made to find an underlying cause (Table 12). Sometimes the history and physical examination will suggest the diagnosis or provide a guide to relevant investigations. Chronic bronchitis and emphysema and chronic alcoholism are usually readily diagnosed from the history. Bronchial carcinoma, foreign body and bronchiectasis should be suspected if pneumonia repeatedly involves the same part of the lung, and relevant investigations include bronchoscopy or bronchography. Oesophageal lesions such as stricture or achalasia may be diagnosed by barium swallow. Peripheral blood examination, serum electrophoresis and bone marrow examination assist

Table 12 Causes of recurrent pneumonia

Chronic bronchitis and emphysema
Bronchial carcinoma
Bronchiectasis
Foreign body
Chronic alcoholism
Oesophageal lesions
Multiple myeloma
Leukaemia
Lymphoma
Cystic fibrosis
Allergic bronchopulmonary aspergillosis

in the diagnosis of multiple myeloma and other immunological disorders. Cysticic fibrosis is a cause of recurrent pneumonia in children and teenagers and can be detected by a sweat test. Allergic bronchopulmonary aspergillosis is discussed on page 119.

PREVENTION

Prevention is directed primarily towards avoiding the situations which predispose to pneumonia. Whenever the level of consciousness is impaired it is imperative to take precautions to prevent inhalation of foreign material. This is particularly important in patients recovering from anaesthesia, and such patients must be kept under close observation until they have regained consciousness. Aspiration is unlikely if the patient is nursed on his side. Equipment for bronchial suction must be kept at the bedside because if the patient inhales vomitus there is no time to obtain lifesaving apparatus from elsewhere. Parents must continually educate their children about the dangers of putting small objects in their mouths.

Postoperative pneumonia may be prevented by physiotherapy before and after surgery, and is essential in patients with chronic bronchitis. Regular postural drainage and prophylactic antibiotics reduce the risk of pneumonia in bronchiectasis. The patient with chronic bronchitis should start tetracycline or ampicillin at the first sign of an upper respiratory tract infection and this may also be indicated in other chronic conditions which predispose to pneumonia.

NON-INFECTIVE PNEUMONIAS

Pneumonias which are not due to infection are uncommon.

Allergic pneumonias: pulmonary eosinophilia
Allergic pneumonias represent a hypersensitivity reaction and are a form of pulmonary eosinophilia. The characteristic picture includes recurrent pulmonary infiltrations, cough, wheeze, fever and eosinophilia of the peripheral blood (p. 245).

Chemical pneumonias
Lipoid pneumonia
Inhalation of oil may cause lipoid pneumonia in persons who regularly use oily nose drops or laxatives containing liquid paraffin. Lipoid pneumonia does not cause the typical symptoms of an infective pneumonia and is usually detected radiographically. It causes

a localized dense opacity in the lower lobe resembling carcinoma and its true nature is determined only after resection.

Pneumonia due to petrol or kerosene

Petrol or kerosene may be ingested accidently by children, especially when they are stored in old lemonade or coca-cola bottles. Parents should be aware that this habit can have a fatal outcome. If vomiting occurs, the petrol or kerosene may be inhaled and cause broncho-pneumonia. Gastric lavage must not be carried out, but oxygen and corticosteroids should be given. Inhalation of petrol fumes may occur in workers in the petroleum industry and causes pulmonary oedema, neurological symptoms and pneumonia.

Mendelson's syndrome

This is a rare condition in which inhalation of acid gastric contents during or immediately after general anaesthesia causes acute pulmonary oedema and acute airways' obstruction. It is not strictly a form of pneumonia but is included here for convenience. Treatment includes antibiotics and oxygen.

Radiation pneumonia

Pneumonia may follow radiotherapy to the chest but with improved techniques it is now uncommon. The pneumonia develops about 4 weeks after a course of radiotherapy, and should be suspected if the patient becomes breathless and the chest radiograph shows shadowing which is maximal in the mid zones. Corticosteroids are given for several months to relieve breathlessness and to reduce fibrosis.

FURTHER READING

Calder M A, McHardy V U, Schonell M E 1970 Importance of pneumococcal typing in pneumonia. Lancet i:5

Crofton J, Douglas A 1981 Respiratory diseases. 3rd edn. Blackwell, Oxford

Lancet Editorial 1983 How common is Legionnaire's Disease? Lancet I:103

MacFarlane J T, Ward M J, Finch R G, Macrae A D 1982 Hospital study of adult community-acquired pneumonia. Lancet ii:255

McHardy V U, Schonell M E 1972 Ampicillin dosage and use of prednisolone in the treatment of pneumonia: cooperative controlled trial. British Medical Journal 4:569

Schonell M E, Gray W, Moffat M A J, Calder M A, Stewart S M 1969 The relationship between the aetiology of pneumonia in adults and certain clinical and radiographic findings. British Journal of Diseases of the Chest 63:140

White R J, Blainey A D, Harrison K Joy, Clarke S K R 1981 Causes of pneumonia presenting to a district general hospital. Thorax 36:566

9

Commonest cause is 2° to bronc Ca.

Lung abscess and empyema

LUNG ABSCESS

Definition
A lung abscess is a localized area of pulmonary suppuration and necrosis with a central cavity, caused by infection with pyogenic organisms.

Epidemiology
The incidence of lung abscess has fallen considerably since improved methods of anaesthesia have reduced the risk of postoperative inhalation, and antibiotics have been available to treat acute respiratory infections. However, the incidence of lung abscess secondary to bronchial carcinoma has increased, and in Britain this is now the commonest cause.

Aetiology, pathogenesis, pathology
Lung abscess may be caused by a variety of bacteria including *Staph. aureus, Str. pneumoniae, K. pneumoniae, H. influenzae, Proteus, Pseudomonas, E. coli* and anaerobic bacteria. Often no pathogens are isolated because the patient has had previous antibiotic treatment. Bacteria reach the lung principally through the bronchial tree or the bloodstream and less frequently through the chest wall or the diaphragm.

Lung abscess is usually secondary to bronchial carcinoma, inhalation of foreign material or pneumonia. occ septicaemia
p'y injection, chest wounds.

Bronchial carcinoma
Lung abscess secondary to bronchial carcinoma results from infection of retained secretions distal to the tumour. Bronchial carcinoma should be suspected whenever lung abscess develops in a patient over the age of 40.

Inhalation of foreign material

Conditions which lower the level of consciousness and depress the epiglottic and cough reflexes predispose to inhalation of vomitus or other foreign material. In this context, lung abscess most frequently complicates chronic alcoholism and drug overdose. In the majority of patients gross dental sepsis is present.

Inhaled foreign material is more likely to enter the right lung than the left because the right main bronchus follows more closely the line of the trachea. If aspiration occurs while the patient is lying on his back, foreign material enters the apical segment of the right lower lobe, but if the patient is lying on his side the posterior and apical segments of the upper lobe are involved. These are the common sites of lung abscess secondary to inhalation of foreign material.

Inhaled foreign material acts as a focus of infection and initially causes pneumonia which is often segmental but may involve a whole lobe. Suppuration and necrosis result in abscess formation. Ulceration into the bronchial tree allows drainage of pus, leaving a cavity lined by granulation tissue.

Pneumonia

Lung abscess complicates 2 per cent of all pneumonias. It mainly follows staphylococcal and klebsiella pneumonia, but may complicate pneumonia due to other bacteria if antibiotic treatment has been delayed or if the patient has an immunological disorder. In staphylococcal pneumonia multiple abscesses may develop, and in children these may progressively enlarge due to valvular obstruction of the bronchial communication which allows air to enter the cavity on inspiration but prevents it leaving during expiration. This results in thin walled cysts, pneumatoceles, which may rupture into the pleural space causing pneumothorax or pyopneumothorax. Klebsiella pneumonia may cause large chronic abscesses in the upper lobes, especially in alcoholics.

Septicaemia, pulmonary infarction and *chest wounds* are occasionally complicated by lung abscess.

Clinical features

The earliest manifestations of lung abscess are fever, cough, pleuritic pain and malaise. When bronchial drainage is established haemoptysis may occur and copious purulent sputum is expectorated. Lung abscess should be suspected if these symptoms follow any situation which predisposes to inhalation of foreign material. Severe systemic upset, persistent fever and weight loss occur when treatment is delayed.

Lung abscess secondary to pneumonia causes symptoms which appear 2 to 3 weeks after the onset of the illness. Recurrence of fever, increased purulent sputum, malaise and haemoptysis occur at a stage when the patient would normally be expected to be recovering.

Physical examination. Finger clubbing may develop within a few weeks in patients with lung abscess. Clubbing should also suggest the possibility of an underlying bronchial carcinoma. The percussion note and breath sounds may be decreased if the abscess is large, but often there are no abnormal signs.

Investigations

Chest radiograph. Lung abscess initially causes a localized homogeneous opacity, but after bronchial drainage is established and pus is expectorated a cavity with a fluid level appears (Fig. 12). This is the typical appearance of a lung abscess. In 85 per cent of cases secondary to inhalation the abscess is in the upper lobe or in the apical segment of the lower lobe.

Sputum examination. Several specimens of sputum are examined for bacteria, including *M. tuberculosis* and anaerobes. Isolation of *Staph. aureus* or *Str. pneumoniae* in moderate numbers is usually aetiologically significant. Gram negative bacteria are of doubtful significance unless they are isolated in heavy growth on more than one occasion. Sputum should always be examined for malignant cells.

Blood culture. This is done in all cases and if bacteria are isolated it is probable that they are playing a causal role.

Peripheral blood. Leucocytosis occurs in 50 per cent of patients.

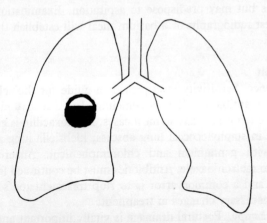

Fig. 12 Lung abscess. The differential diagnosis of a cavitated lesion includes tuberculosis and cavitated bronchial carcinoma.

Bronchoscopy. This is often necessary to exclude bronchial obstruction by carcinoma or foreign body and is mandatory in heavy smokers because of the likelihood of tumour. A normal bronchoscopy does not completely exclude carcinoma because the tumour may lie beyond bronchoscopic vision.

Differential diagnosis

Bronchial carcinoma. A bronchial carcinoma may cavitate if the centre of the tumour becomes necrotic because of inadequate blood supply. The walls of the cavity are composed of tumour and are frequently thick and irregular. Cavitated bronchial carcinoma often causes haemoptysis but it may be symptomless. Bronchial carcinoma should be suspected in any person over the age of 40 who presents with a solitary cavitated pulmonary lesion.

Pulmonary tuberculosis. Usually the patient gives a history of cough, weight loss and ill health of several months duration. Acid fast bacilli are usually present in the sputum and the tuberculin test is positive. Tuberculous cavities are often multiple and bilateral and do not contain fluid levels.

Infected emphysematous bulla. A large emphysematous bulla sometimes becomes infected and appears in the chest radiograph as an apparent 'cavity' with a fluid level which may be indistinguishable from a lung abscess. Differentiation is easy if previous radiographs show bullae at the same site.

Hiatus hernia. A large hiatus hernia may simulate the radiographic appearance of a lung abscess by causing an apparent fluid level behind the heart. Hiatus hernia itself does not cause respiratory symptoms but may predispose to aspiration. Examination of previous chest radiographs or a barium meal will establish the correct diagnosis.

Treatment

Antibiotics. Sensitivity tests provide a guide for the selection of appropriate antibiotics. Benzyl penicillin, 1 to 2 mega units bd, by I. M. injection is effective in most cases. Flucloxacillin is given with penicillin in staphylococcal lung abscess; klebsiella lung abscess is treated with gentamicin and chloramphenicol. Anaerobes will respond to metronidazole. Antibiotics must be continued for at least 6 weeks, and a common error is to stop treatment too soon or to make unnecessary changes in treatment.

Physiotherapy. Postural drainage is vitally important and hastens resolution.

Surgery. Resection may be necessary if the abscess has not decreased in size after antibiotic treatment for 4 to 6 weeks. Resection is carried out in patients with suspected or proven bronchial carcinoma.

Prognosis
Prognosis depends on the underlying cause. Lung abscess secondary to bronchial carcinoma has a poor prognosis. Lung abscess due to inhalation or pneumonia is rarely fatal. Involvement of the pleura may result in empyema or pyopneumothorax but both are uncommon. Cerebral abscess and amyloid disease are rare complications of lung abscess.

Prevention
Lung abscess can often be prevented if precautions are taken to avoid inhalation of secretions and vomitus in patients whose level of consciousness is impaired. Bronchoscopy is often necessary if inhalation occurs after anaesthesia or drug overdose. Pneumonia is rarely complicated by lung abscess if treated promptly and adequately with antibiotics.

EMPYEMA

Definition
Empyema is the term used to describe a purulent pleural effusion. The pus may lie in the general pleural space or may be loculated (encysted empyema). Empyema may be acute or chronic and is invariably unilateral.

Aetiology, pathogenesis, pathology
Infection reaches the pleural space through the bronchial tree, the bloodstream or the chest wall. Empyema is usually secondary to *pneumonia, lung abscess, bronchiectasis* or *tuberculosis*. Since the discovery of antibiotics empyema has become a rare complication of these diseases. Empyema is an occasional complication of penetrating chest wounds.

Initially the pus in the pleural space is thin but it rapidly becomes thick due to accumulation of fibrin and disintegrated leucocytes. The visceral and parietal pleura are covered with fibrinous exudate and the pus may become encysted by adhesions. A loculated empyema usually lies between the lung and the chest wall.

The pus within an empyema is under tension and if untreated it may rupture through the chest wall or into a bronchus causing a bronchopleural fistula and pyopneumothorax.

Resolution of an empyema is achieved by aspiration or drainage of the pus so that the lung re-expands. If the empyema is not treated promptly it becomes chronic and layers of fibrin over the visceral pleura prevent re-expansion. Pleural calcification may occur in chronic empyema especially if it is due to tuberculosis.

Clinical features

The clinical features are due to the underlying cause of the empyema, the local effects of fluid in the pleural space and the systemic effects of a collection of pus.

The clinical features of the underlying conditions are discussed in detail elsewhere. Empyema secondary to pneumonia causes recurrence of fever during convalescence; tuberculous empyema is suspected if there is a long history of cough, ill health, night sweats and weight loss.

Fluid in the pleural space causes breathlessness, cough and pleuritic pain, but these symptoms are often overshadowed by the systemic symptoms, especially in chronic empyema.

The systemic symptoms include fever, rigors, sweating, malaise, anorexia and weight loss. When these symptoms have been present for several months it can be assumed that the empyema is chronic.

Physical examination. The signs of pleural effusion (p. 229) are present if there is free fluid in the pleural space but these signs are absent when the empyema is encysted. The percussion note and breath sounds may be reduced over an encysted empyema. Finger clubbing may develop within a few weeks and is common in chronic empyema. In chronic empyema the chest wall is flattened and chest movement is greatly reduced. Chronic empyema may cause spinal scoliosis.

Investigations

Chest radiograph. Pus in the general pleural space gives rise to the typical appearance of pleural effusion (Fig. 38). A dense homogeneous opacity obliterates the costophrenic angle and the lower part of the lung. The upper border of the opacity is concave and extends laterally towards the axilla. A large empyema obliterates most of the lung field and causes mediastinal displacement to the opposite side. In chronic empyema the mediastinum may be pulled towards the affected side by fibrosis.

An encysted empyema appears as a localized dense homogeneous opacity which may involve any part of the pleural space but is commonly situated in the lower part of the paravertebral gutter. A lateral radiograph is necessary to determine the exact site of an encysted empyema.

If a bronchopleural fistula develops, air enters the pleural space giving a pyopneumothorax which is recognized by a fluid level. The commonest cause of a fluid level is the accidental entry of air into the pleural space during pleural aspiration.

Pleural aspiration. This is carried out immediately if empyema is suspected and a wide bore needle is inserted at the site of maximum dullness. Aspirations of pus confirms the diagnosis. The pus and also sputum specimens are examined for bacteria including tubercle bacilli.

Differential diagnosis

The differential diagnosis includes other conditions which cause pleural effusion, and diseases which cause marked systemic upset such as lung abscess and tuberculosis. The correct diagnosis is readily established by pleural aspiration.

Treatment

Pleural aspiration. Prompt aspiration of the pus is essential and must be continued until the empyema space is dry. Early in the disease thin pus can be removed by repeated needle aspiration or by insertion of an intercostal catheter with underwater seal drainage. If the patient is seen more than a month after onset of symptoms limited thoracotomy is usually necessary to obtain adequate drainage.

Antibiotics. The choice of antibiotics is influenced by the results of sensitivity tests. If bacteria are not isolated a combination of I. M. benzyl penicillin, 1 mega unit bd, gentamycin, 80 mg I. M. t.d.s., and metronidazole 400 mg orally t.d.s. is usually effective. Flucloc-acillin is combined with penicillin in staphylococcal empyema. Antibiotics must be continued for six weeks. Tuberculous empyema is treated with triple chemotherapy.

Surgery. It is usually necessary resect a chronic empyema and to carry out decortication of the lung in order to obtain re-expansion.

Cerebral abscess and amyloid disease are rare complications of empyema.

FURTHER READING

Barnett T B, Herring C L 1971 Lung abscess, initial and late results of medical treatment. Archives of Internal Medicine 127:217

Benfield G F A 1981 Recent trends in empyema thoracis. British Journal of Disease of the Chest 75:358

Leading article 1970 Non-specific lung abscess. British Medical Journal 3:120

Flavell G 1966 Lung abscess. British Medical Journal i:1032

10

Bronchial obstruction and pulmonary collapse

Definition
Complete obstruction of a large bronchus is followed by absorption of the air in the lung tissue supplied by the bronchus and collapse of the affected lung, lobe or segment.

Aetiology
Pulmonary collapse may be due to occlusion of the lumen of the bronchus or external compression of the bronchus. The most important causes of bronchial obstruction are:

1. *Bronchial carcinoma.*
2. *Inhalation of foreign material.* Children are liable to inhale small objects such as peanuts, stones or coins, while adults are likely to inhale vomitus during anaesthesia or alcoholic intoxication.
3. *Retained secretions.* After thoracic and abdominal surgery coughing is painful and retained secretions may cause *post-operative pulmonary collapse*, especially in patients with chronic bronchitis. Ineffective cough in neuromuscular disorders and in debilitated patients also predisposes to retention of bronchial secretions. In *asthma, allergic bronchopulmonary aspergillosis, whooping cough, measles* and *pneumonia*, plugs of viscous mucus may cause bronchial obstruction.

Pathology and functional abnormality
Complete bronchial obstruction causes pulmonary collapse and the airless lung contracts towards the hilum. The mediastinum is drawn towards the side of the collapse and the hemidiaphragm is elevated on the same side. The remaining aerated lung tissue expands to fill the space normally occupied by the collapsed lung. This is termed *compensatory emphysema*. Collapsed lung acts as a physiological shunt and mixed venous blood passes directly into the systemic circulation producing hypoxaemia if the collapse is extensive. Compensatory hyperventilation prevents carbon dioxide retention.

Partial bronchial obstruction allows air to enter the lung during inspiration but may prevent air leaving the lung during expiration if the normal expiratory narrowing of the bronchi is sufficient to cause complete bronchial obstruction. This causes overdistension of the lung supplied by the partially obstructed bronchus and is called *obstructive emphysema*. During expiration the mediastinum moves towards the opposite side because the pressure in the affected lung is greater than in the contralateral lung. The mediastinal swing can be seen on fluoroscopic screening.

Complete or partial bronchial obstruction prevents drainage of bronchial secretions. and predisposes to bacterial infection which may cause *pneumonia* or *lung abscess*. If the obstruction persists *bronchiectasis* may develop.

Clinical features

The clinical features of pulmonary collapse depend on the extent of the collapse and the underlying cause. The main symptoms are breathlessness and cough. These are often sudden in onset and may be preceded by a choking sensation if the obstruction is due to inhalation of foreign material. Postoperative collapse causes cough and fever which develop on the second or third postoperative day. Segmental collapse may not give rise to symptoms or signs and usually it can only be detected radiographically.

Physical examination. The pulse and respiratory rate are increased and central cyanosis may be present. The chest wall is flattened and chest movement is reduced on the affected side. The trachea and apex beat are displaced towards the side of the lesion. The percussion note is dull and the breath sounds are reduced or absent over the collapsed lung. Bronchial breathing may be heard if the obstruction is incomplete so that air enters the affected lung. Compensatory emphysema and obstructive emphysema do not cause physical signs.

Investigations

Chest radiograph. Lobar collapse produces a homogeneous opacity which is limited by the fissures of the lung and has a characteristic shape (Figs. 13 to 16). Collapse of the whole lung causes a homogeneous opacity which occupies the hemithorax. The trachea and heart shadow are displaced towards the affected side and the hemidiaphragm is elevated. The other causes of a homogeneous opacity include lobar pneumonia, which does not cause mediastinal displacement, and pleural effusion, which causes mediastinal displacement to the opposite side if it is large.

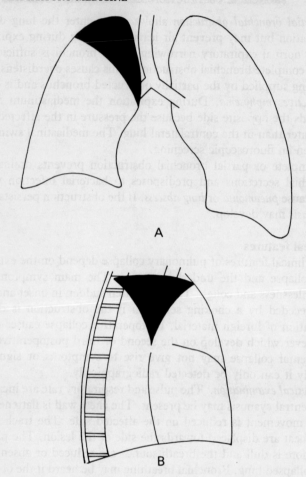

Fig. 13 Collapse of the right upper lobe. (a) PA view; (b) Lateral view.

The homogeneous opacity is limited on its inferior aspect by the horizontal fissure which is pulled upwards. The trachea and heart are displaced towards the side of the collapse and the right hemidiaphragm is elevated.

Bronchoscopy. Usually bronchoscopy is necessary to determine the cause of the bronchial obstruction; bronchial biopsy often confirms the diagnosis if bronchial carcinoma is responsible.

Differential diagnosis
The differential diagnosis includes other conditions which cause sudden breathlessness such as acute bronchial asthma, pulmonary embolism, spontaneous pneumothorax and acute pulmonary

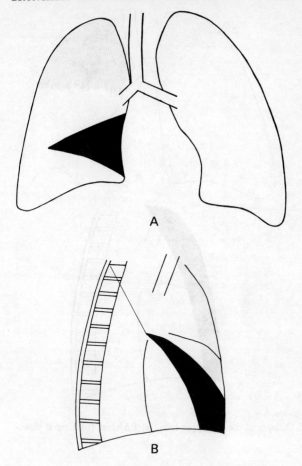

Fig. 14 Collapse of the middle lobe. (a) PA view; (b) Lateral view.

The homogeneous opacity is limited on its superior aspect by the horizontal fissure which is pulled down. The trachea and heart are displaced towards the side of the collapse and the right hemidiaphragm is elevated.

oedema. Postoperative collapse must be differentiated from pneumonia and pulmonary infarction.

Treatment

Pulmonary collapse due to inhalation of foreign matter or retained secretions is treated by intensive physiotherapy, which includes postural drainage, chest percussion and assited coughing. If the lung does not re-expand within a few hours, bronchoscopic aspiration is carried out. Emergency bronchoscopy may be necessary to relieve

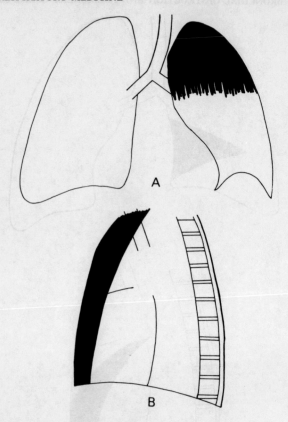

Fig. 15 Collapse of the left upper lobe. (a) PA view; (b) Lateral view.

collapse which is causing acute respiratory distress. Oxygen is given if the patient is hypoxaemic and antibiotics given to control infection. Collapse due to bronchial carcinoma is treated by surgery or radiotherapy.

Prevention
Physiotherapy before and after surgery will usually prevent postoperative pulmonary collapse and is essential in patients with chronic bronchitis. In these patients respiratory function should be assessed before surgery by carrying out ventilation tests and blood gas analysis. Smoking should always be forbidden before surgery. General anaesthesia is best avoided in anyone with an acute respiratory infection except in an emergency.

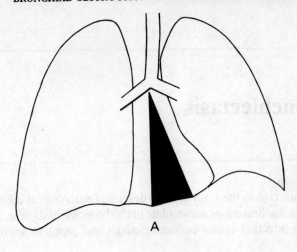

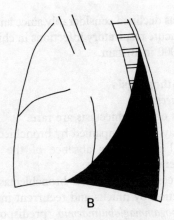

Fig. 16 Collapse of the left lower lobe. (a) PA view; (b) Lateral view.

The homogeneous opacity is obscured by the heart shadow but is recognized by the appearance of the oblique fissure which forms a straight line passing downwards from the hilum to the diaphragm.

11

Bronchiectasis

Definition
Bronchiectasis is the term used to described pathological dilation of the bronchi. Secretions accumulate in the bronchiectasis bronchi and chronic infection causes persistent cough and purulent sputum.

Epidemiology
The prevalence has declined considerably since antibiotics have been available to treat acute respiratory infections in childhood and is now less than 1 per 1000 in Britain.

Aetiology and pathogenesis
Congenital bronchiectasis
Congenital causes of bronchiectasis are rare.

Dextrocardia may be accompanied by bronchiectasis and if associated with frontal sinusitis or absence of the frontal sinuses is known as Kartagener's syndrome.

Cystic fibrosis commonly causes bronchiectasis as a result of bronchial obstruction by mucus and recurrent infections.

Congenital hypogammaglobulinaemia predisposes to recurrent pneumonia which may give rise to bronchiectasis. Acquired immunological disorders are unlikely to cause bronchiectasis because death occurs before permanent bronchial dilation develops.

Acquired bronchiectasis
Bronchial obstruction and *bacterial infection* are the two main factors responsible for bronchiectasis. Obstruction of lobar, segmental or smaller bronchi results in collapse of the lung supplied by the obstructed bronchi (Fig. 17). Secretions accumulate distal to the obstruction, and if this is not relieved promptly the secretions become infected. Inflammation of the bronchial wall causes destruction of the elastic and muscular tissue which is followed by weakening and eventually dilatation of the bronchi. Secretions are not properly cleared from the bronchiectatic bronchi and chronic infec-

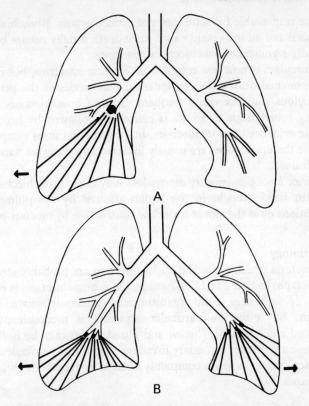

Fig. 17 Pathogensis of bronchiectasis. (a) Obstruction of a large proximal bronchus; (b) Obstruction of multiple small bronchi. Obstruction causes pulmonary collapse, and infection of retained secretions damages the bronchial walls which dilate as a result of inspiratory expansile forces.

tion develops. In the early stages the bronchi may return to normal if the obstruction is removed and infection has not caused irreversible damage.

There are numerous theories concerning the mechanism which causes the bronchial dilation and the exact site at which it acts. It seems probable that one of the forces responsible is the repeated negative inspiratory pressure acting on the weakened bronchial wall.

Whooping cough, measles and *pneumonia* in early childhood are the most common conditions leading to bronchiectasis. In these diseases viscous sputum is likely to cause obstruction of multiple small bronchi. Bronchiectasis begins in childhood because the bronchi are small and relatively easily occluded; respiratory infections in adults are unlikely to give rise to bronchiectasis.

Foreign bodies or *bronchial adenoma* may obstruct larger bronchi and are responsible for some cases of bronchiectasis. Bronchial carcinoma is not an important cause since death usually occurs before clinically significant bronchiectasis develops.

Tuberculosis is now less common in Western countries, but in the past bronchial obstruction by enlarged hilar nodes of the primary tuberculous complex was a frequent cause of bronchiectasis. Pulmonary tuberculosis in adults is commonly followed by bronchographic evidence of bronchiectasis, but this rarely causes symptoms because the upper lobes are usually involved and these are naturally well drained.

Allergic bronchopulmonary aspergillosis may cause bronchiectasis of medium sized bronchi in the region affected by the pulmonary infiltrations or at the site of bronchial obstruction by mucous plugs.

Bacteriology

The bacteria which cause the initial infection are probably streptococci, staphylococci and *H. influenzae*. Once bronchiectasis is established, *H. influenzae* is the organism most commonly isolated from sputum, but often no particular organism is predominant. In advanced cases *E. coli*, *Proteus* and *Pseudomonas* may be isolated, but these are usually secondary invaders of doubtful aetiological significance. *Staph. aureus* is commonly isolated from patients with cystic fibrosis.

Pathology and functional abnormality

Bronchiectasis may be localized or widespread. The left lung is affected more often than the right, although in 50 per cent of cases bronchiectasis is bilateral. The commonest sites are the lower lobes, the lingula and the middle lobe. This distribution is determined by the less efficient drainage of secretions from the lower bronchi.

In advanced bronchiectasis the bronchi are grossly dilated and filled with pus. The mucosa is replaced by granulation tissue and the elastic and muscle tissue destroyed. The bronchi are crowded together and the segment or lobe becomes fibrotic and contracted. Large anastomoses develop between the bronchial and pulmonary arteries and this is responsible for the relatively severe haemoptysis which may occur in bronchiectasis.

The degree of functional impairment in bronchiectasis is related to the extent of the disease. In severe cases the affected lung is sufficiently underventilated and underperfused to contribute little to gas exchange. Bronchiectasis is commonly accompanied by chronic bronchitis.

Consideration of the pathology readily explains the clinical features and the natural course of the disease.

Clinical features

Onset. Symptoms usually begin in childhood. In 75 per cent of cases symptoms are present by the fifth year and onset can be traced to an attack of whooping cough, measles or pneumonia. Despite this, the diagnosis is often not made until adult life.

Cough and sputum. A history of persistent cough and purulent sputum since childhood is virtually diagnostic of bronchiectasis. Once bronchiectasis has developed the dilated bronchi continue to accumulate purulent secretions and the patient will forever have cough and sputum unless the affected area is resected.

The volume of sputum and the degree of purulence vary; during acute episodes of infection both increase. The volume of sputum varies from 50 to 500 ml/24 hours. Paroxysms of coughing may be precipitated by change in posture which causes secretions to leave the affected bronchi and enter normal bronchi, resulting in stimulation of the cough reflex. For this reason cough and sputum are particularly troublesome on rising in the morning, on exertion and on lying down at night. Rarely bronchiectasis does not cause cough and sputum and is called 'dry' bronchiectasis.

Breathlessness. This is uncommon unless the bronchiectasis is widespread or the patient has associated chronic bronchitis.

Recurrent haemoptysis. Haemoptysis is a common symptom and is usually the result of acute infection. The sputum is stained with fresh blood and occasionally profuse haemoptysis occurs due to bleeding from bronchopulmonary anastomoses.

Recurrent pneumonia and pleurisy. The patient with bronchiectasis commonly gives a history of recurrent attacks of pneumonia and pleurisy, often dating from childhood. These infections may be considered part of the natural history of the disease and characteristically recur at the same site. Occasionally the patient with bronchiectasis first presents with recurrent pneumonia or haemoptysis.

Chronic sinusitis. This is present in 70 per cent of patients.

Systemic symptoms. Widespread bronchiectasis may cause malaise, anorexia, weight loss and fever. These symptoms are due to chronic sepsis and are uncommon if the patient is taking prophylactic chemotherapy. Failure to thrive may occur in children before the diagnosis is established.

Physical examination. The characteristic finding is persistent coarse crepitations which are heard over one or both lower lobes, the middle lobe or lingula. Fibrosis or collapse may cause reduced chest movement, mediastinal displacement, localized dullness on percussion and reduced breath sounds. Finger clubbing occurs in about 50 per cent of patients. Central cyanosis may be present in severe bronchiectasis.

Investigations

Chest radiograph. This may be normal but usually shows patchy shadowing, cystic areas or streaky fibrosis in one or both lower zones. Crowded linear shadows in the lower zones represent thickened bronchial walls. These appearances are suggestive of bronchiectasis but are not diagnostic. Segmental or lobar collapse is sometimes present.

Sputum examination. Sputum culture is carried out at times of acute infection. Gram negative bacteria, with the exception of *H. influenzae*, are of doubtful significance unless isolated repeatedly in heavy growth.

Bronchography. The diagnosis can be confirmed only by bronchography. This shows pooling of contast medium in the dilated bronchi. Bronchography is usually unnecessary in middle-aged or elderly people, since surgery is rarely indicated after the age of 40, and a diagnosis made on clinical grounds is quite acceptable. In younger people bronchography is advisable to establish the diagnosis and plan treatment, but in young children can usually be deferred for some years. A course of antibiotics and physiotherapy before bronchography improves the quality of the bronchograms.

Bronchoscopy. This may be necessary in children and young adults to exclude a foreign body or a benign tumour. It is unnecessary in older people in whom bronchiectasis has been present for many years.

Sweat test, serum immunoglobulins. These estimations are used as screening tests for cystic fibrosis and hypogamma-globulinaemia and should be carried out in all children and young adults with bronchiectasis.

Differential diagnosis

The diagnosis of bronchiectasis is not difficult because cough and sputum since childhood and persistent localized crepitations are unlikely to be mistaken. Bronchiectasis should be suspected in any patient with recurrent haemoptysis or recurrent pneumonia.

Acute bronchitis. Recurrent attacks of acute bronchitis are a common problem in children but may be differentiated from bronchiectasis by the absence of cough and sputum between the episodes of acute infection.

Chronic bronchitis. Cough and sputum do not appear until after the age of 40 and are accompanied by wheeze and rhonchi. The latter are late features of bronchiectasis unless there is associated chronic bronchitis or asthma. Sputum is not as copious in chronic bronchitis and emphysema nor as chronically purulent. When more than one disease is present a careful history and ventilation tests will demonstrate which is the main cause of the patient's sympfoms. If the patient is elderly or has moderate airways obstruction there is little practical value in bronchography since resection is usually contraindicated.

Pneumonia. This should not be confused with bronchiectasis since the cough and sputum will be of recent onset unless the pneumonia is a complication of bronchiectasis or chronic bronchitis.

Pulmonary tuberculosis; bronchial carcinoma. These diseases cause chronic cough and haemoptysis but can usually be differentiated from bronchiectasis by a detailed history, a chest radiograph and sputum examination for tubercle bacilli and malignant cells. Bronchoscopy is carried out if bronchial carcinoma cannot be excluded with certainty.

Treatment
The essentials of treatment are postural drainage, physiotherapy and prompt antibiotics for exacerbations of infection. Postural drainage produces relief from embarrassing cough and expectoration, while prompt chemotherapy reduces sputum volume and purulence during an exacerbation.

Postural drainage. The patient is instructed how to carry out postural drainage of the affected lobes. This can be achieved by raising the foot of the bed or in young patients by lying over the side of the bed. Postural drainage should be done for 20 minutes on waking and before retiring. Constant encouragement is necessary, otherwise postural drainage is neglected because it is time consuming during the morning 'rush hour' and frustrating during the evening leisure hours. Invariably patients feel the benefit of regular postural draining. It is particularly important during episodes of acute infection. Spouses or other relatives should be taught how to give simple physiotherapy and to do this once or twice daily.

Antibiotics. Acute exacerbations of infection are usually treated with ampicillin, 250 mg 6-hourly. Antibiotics are continued for 1 to 2 weeks. Patients who have frequent exacerbations will usually benefit from prophylactic antibiotics given throughout the winter, or all year round if necessary. Oxytetracycline 500 mg bd, doxycycline 100 mg once daily or sulphametopyrazine 2 g once weekly are effective.

Associated sinusitis, asthma or respiratory failure require appropriate treatment. Smoking should be prohibited.

Surgery. Surgery is indicated in patients under the age of 40 with persistent troublesome symptoms due to localized bronchiectasis. In children surgery is best deferred until the early teens because spontaneous improvement may occur. Preoperative bronchograms of good quality are essential to localize the extent of the disease. In patients with localized bronchiectasis the results of surgery are excellent and freedom from symptoms can transform the patient's life. The usual operation is segmental resection or lobectomy. Surgery will not relieve symptoms if residual areas of bronchiectasis remain, and for these reasons is rarely indicated in widespread disease. Associated irreversible airways obstruction of moderate severity contraindicates surgery.

Complications and prognosis

Recurrent haemoptysis, pneumonia and *pleurisy* are common and frequently follow an upper respiratory tract infection. They should be treated promptly with ampicillin. Rarely, haemoptysis is life-threatening and emergency resection is necessary. *Empyema, lung abcess, cerebral abscess* and *amyloid disease* are rare complications.

With skilled medical and surgical care most patients lead a normal life, although a small percentage have progressive symptoms and die from *respiratory failure* and *cor pulmonale.*

Prevention

Bronchiectasis can be largely prevented if acute lower respiratory tract infections in children are treated with antibiotics and physiotherapy. If pulmonary collapse occurs it must be relieved promptly. It is wise for children and young adults to have a chest radiograph after any severe respiratory infection to ensure that there are no residual abnormalities.

FURTHER READING

Borrie J, Lichter I 1965 Surgical treatment of bronchiectasis: ten year survey. British Medical Journal ii:908

British Medical Journal 1975 Bronchiectasis today. British Medical Journal Leading article iv 604

British Medical Journal 1979 Bronchiectasis, congenital and acquired. British Medical Journal Leading article i:1380–1381

Clarke N S 1963 Bronchiectasis in childhood. British Medical Journal, i:80

Crofton J 1966 Diagnosis and treatment of bronchiectasis. British Medical Journal i:721

12

Bronchial asthma

Definition
Bronchial asthma is characterized by recurrent, paroxysmal attacks of wheezing due to generalised airways obstruction which changes in severity over short periods of time either spontaneously or as a result of treatment. Sometimes asthma is chronic and there is persistent airways obstruction.

Epidemiology
About 5 to 10 per cent of children suffer from asthma, while among adults the prevalence is about 3 to 5 per cent. In children asthma is twice as common in boys and girls but in adults it is slightly more common in women. Asthma may begin at any age but in over 50 per cent of cases the disease first appears in childhood, often before five years of age.

The mortality rate from asthma is about 2 per 100 000. Failure to recognise severity by patients, relatives and doctors can cause delay in starting appropriate treatment and may also lead to underprescribing of corticosteroids and bronchodilators.

AETIOLOGY AND PATHOGENESIS

In patients with asthma the bronchial tree is *hyper-reactive* and a variety of stimuli may precipitate airways obstruction. Allergy and respiratory infections are the commonest factors which precipitate acute asthma but their relative importance varies in different individuals and in different countries. In the majority of patients, an asthma attack may be triggered off by one of a number of factors, and often it is impossible to determine the factor responsible for a particular attack.

Allergy
Inhaled allergens The commonest allergens which cause asthma are house dust mite, grass and flower pollens, dander from cats, dogs

and horses, and feathers. Most asthmatics are very allergic to house dust and the antigen in the dust which is mainly responsible is derived from the house dust mite *Dermatophagoides*. The mite lives in bedding and mattresses, particulary in damp rooms and feeds on scales of keratin shed from the human skin. Other inhaled allergens which may cause asthma include fungi such as *A. fumigatus* (p. 119).

Ingested allergens These play a less important role, but milk, chocolate, eggs, fish and alcohol occasionally produce asthma. Drugs such as aspirin, penicillin and iodides may also precipitate asthma attacks. Aspirin asthma is a serious harzard in patients with nasal polyps and asthma.

Allergy is mainly responsible for asthma in children and young adults and often the attacks have a seasonal or diurnal prevalence. Asthma due to pollen allergy occurs predominantly in the spring and summer while asthma due to fungi develops mainly in the autumn. Nocturnal attacks of asthma may be attributed to allergy to house dust mite or to feather pillows.

Immunological mechanism.
Allergic asthma develops predominantly in atopic individuals who have a constitutional predisposition to become allergic to multiple allergens. If a previously sensitized person inhales an allergen a hypersensitivity reaction occurs in the bronchial tree resulting in an attack of asthma. This reaction begins within minutes of exposure to the allergen and is a type 1 hyersensitivity reaction, mediated by antibodies of the IgE class. In a sensitized individual these antibodies become attached to the cells of the respiratory tract, especially mast cells, and further exposure to the allergen results in an antigen-antibody reaction. The antigen-antibody reaction causes degranulation of the mast cells which release pharmacologically active substances which cause bronchial constriction. There is evidence to show that adenyl cyclase and cyclic adenosine monophosphate are involved in the mast cell reaction.

Knowledge of the nature and role of the pharmacological mediators responsible for the bronchial constriction is incomplete. Histamine, slow-reacting substance A, kinins, prostaglandin and 5-hyroxytryptamine may be involved and probably act by causing bronchial muscle contraction, increased capillary permeability, mucosal oedema and mucus hypersecretion.

In patients with allergic asthma, bronchial challenge with allergens will produce immediate airways obstruction and prick skin tests produce immediate weal and flare reactions. The levels of serum IgE in patients with allergic asthma are higher than the levels in normal individuals and patients with non-allergic asthma.

Individuals who develop allergic asthma have often had infantile eczema and commonly suffer from hay fever and urticaria. In 50 per cent of cases there is a family history of asthma, hay fever or eczema.

Occupational asthma.

Occasionally asthma develops as a result of occupational exposure to certain organic dusts. *Cedar dust asthma* occurs in workers in the wood industry who are exposed to the dust of Canadian Western red cedar. Workers concerned with the manufacture of proteolytic washing powders may develop wheeze, cough and rhinorrhoea after inhalation of enzymes of *B. subtilis* used in the manufacture of washing powders. Toluene disocyanate (TDI) is another cause of industrial asthma. Unlike other forms of allergic asthma, symptoms usually begin 4 to 6 hours after exposure.

Infection

Respiratory infection commonly precipitates acute asthma, particularly in children and middle-aged people. This is probably due to bronchial inflammation which causes narrowing of the airways as a result of mucosal oedema and increased secretions. Alternatively, or in addition, it may be an allergic response to bacterial antigens. The former explanation would seem to apply to many cases of childhood asthma because it often disappears at 12 to 14 years of age. This coincides with rapid increase in growth at puberty and the associated increase in bronchial diameter so that the airways are less easily occluded by inflammation. The agents responsible for respiratory infection in asthma are mainly *Str. pneumoniae*, *H. influenzae* and viruses. Asthma precipitated by infection occurs mainly during the winter.

Exercise-induced asthma

Exercise makes asthma worse because of the increased ventilatory requirements but in some patients exercise is the only factor which precipitates attacks. Exercise-induced asthma is more common in active young individuals, and is probably caused by airway cooling. It may be prevented by inhalation of a bronchodilator or sodium cromoglycate before exercise.

Non-specific stimuli

Changes in temperature and humidity may also precipitate airways obstruction in the asthmatic. Patients with asthma are particularly sensitive to cigarette smoke and often complain that it causes wheeze and chest tightness. Asthmatics rarely smoke, or if they are smokers they invariably stop smoking when they develop asthma.

Beta-blockers, even the 'cardioselective' agents, can precipitate wheezing in asthmatic patients and/or render treatment of attacks more difficult. Fatalities have occurred among asthmatics given B-blockers.

Psychological factors

Emotional stress may aggravate or even precipitate acute asthma but this is rarely an important aetiological factor. Asthmatic patients are surprisingly stable and stoical considering the extremely unpleasant nature of the disease.

Extrinsic and intrinsic asthma

Asthma is sometimes divided into extrinsic and intrinsic types on the basis of the immunological status of the patient and the factors which precipitate acute attacks. The term 'extrinsic asthma' is applied to cases in which the asthma is due to extrinsic allergens. These individuals are usually atopic, with raised IgE levels and positive immediate skin tests to common allergens such as house dust mite. They often have a family history of asthma, eczema, hay fever or urticaria. Extrinsic asthma commonly begins in childhood. In contrast the term 'intrinsic asthma' is used for patients without these features and in whom there are no obvious allergic precipitating factors. Intrinsic asthma often begins in middle age. In practice these terms are of little value because many patients show features of both extrinsic and intrinsic types.

PATHOLOGY AND FUNCTIONAL ABNORMALITY

Airways obstruction is caused by excessive bronchial secretions, oedema of the bronchial mucosa and contraction of bronchial muscle. In fatal asthma tenacious secretions may form viscous casts in the smaller bronchi. There is increase in the number of goblet cells and mucous glands. The bronchial wall is infiltrated with eosinophils and the bronchial muscle is hypertrophied. Asthma does not cause emphysema.

The airways obstruction causes increased resistance to air flow which is responsbile for the wheeze. Wheeze is most marked in expiration because during this phase of respiration the bronchi normally become narrower and shorter. Ventilatory function tests show an obstructive ventilatory defect. Less severe degrees of airways obstruction may be detected by a body plethysmograph. As a result of the airways obstruction there is increase in the work of breathing.

Airways obstruction causes hyperinflation of the lungs with increase in TLC. During an acute attack the resting expiratory level may rise so that the volume of air in the lungs at this point, the FRC, is greatly increased. Residual volume (RV) is also increased. The airways obstruction is relieved by bronchodilator drugs and corticosteroids. Sometimes clinical improvement occurs without improvement in FEV_1 and this may be due to reduction in FRC and RV.

The airways narrowing is not uniform and causes uneven distribution of the inspired air and ventilation-perfusion imbalance. This results in hypoxaemia. Compensatory hyperventilation produces a fall in P_aCO_2. In severe status asthmaticus, in addition to profound hypoxaemia, the P_aCO_2 may rise as a result of hypoventilation due to retention of copious viscous bronchial secretions.

Lung scans in acute asthma show local perfusion defects from pulmonary vasoconstriction due to focal hypoxia or interference with local blood flow by overdistended lung. Acute asthma may cause an increase in pulmonary artery pressure, but right ventricular failure is rare, probably because the airways obstruction is intermittent.

CLINICAL FEATURES

Paroxysmal attacks of wheeze and breathlessness of *sudden onset* are the main symptoms. The attack may be preceded by respiratory infection or exposure to an allergen. Nocturnal wheeze which wakes the patient from sleep is common, particularly in children with house dust mite hypersensitivity. The severity of the wheeze and breathlessness is variable, but commonly both are severe and cause extreme distress.

Chest tightness and *cough* often accompany the wheeze and may be the earliest and sometimes the only symptoms. The cough may be dry or productive of sticky mucoid sputum. The sputum may be purulent if infection is present but occasionally yellow sputum is due to large numbers of eosinophils.

Physical examination. The respiratory rate and the depth of breathing are increased and the patient sits up and leans forward using the accessory muscles of respiration. Audible expiratory wheeze is often the main physical finding.

The pulse is rapid and the degree of tachycardia is an index of the severity of the attack. The chest is hyperinflated and on percussion the upper level of the liver dullness is below the 6th rib in the right midclavicular line. Inspiratory and expiratory rhonchi are heard over both lungs and expiration is prolonged. Pulsus paradoxus may be present.

Usually the acute wheeze lasts for several hours and is then followed by less severe wheeze which persists for some days. Symptoms resolve promptly if treatment is started early.

Clinical types

The clinical course and severity of asthma is variable and it is useful to distinguish the following clinical types.

Episodic asthma

Acute attacks occurs several times a year and between attacks the patient is free from wheeze. The prognosis is good but some patients suffer attacks with increasing frequency and eventually develop chronic asthma.

Status asthmaticus

This is the name given to a severe acute attack of asthma which has been present for some hours. *The following signs indicate severe asthma:* inability of the patient to speak because of breathlessness, central cyanosis, anxiety and restlessness, disturbance of the level of consciousness, retention of large amounts of bronchial secretions, a pulse rate greater than 130/min, pulsus paradoxus, severe chest hyperinflation, barely audible breath sounds and absence of rhonchi. Central cyanosis, anxiety and restlessness are caused by severe hypoxaemia; impaired consciousness is due to hypercapnia; pulsus paradoxus results from pulmonary overinflation, and decreased intensity of the breath sounds indicates severe reduction of tidal volume.

Chronic asthma

The patient with chronic asthma has fairly constant low-grade wheeze and acute attacks are commonly precipitated by respiratory infection. Chronic asthma often begins in middle-aged people without a previous history of asthma. Chronic asthma has a worse prognosis than episodic asthma.

Childhood asthma

Asthma in childhood may be preceded by infantile eczema, the eczema-asthma syndrome. Allergy is a more common precipitating factor in childhood asthma than in asthma of late onset. Respiratory infections also commonly precipitate asthma attacks in children. Chronic asthma in childhood may cause chest deformities such as Harrison's sulcus and pigeon chest. Chronic asthma also impairs growth. Childhood asthma has a good prognosis and only a minority of patients have persistent symptoms in later life.

Allergic bronchopulmonary aspergillosis

This is a form of pulmonary eosinophilia due to hypersensitivity to *A. fumigatus*. It is due to combined type 1 and 3 hypersensitivity reactions and occurs predominantly in atopic people. It is characterized by episodic wheeze, migratory pulmonary infiltrations and eosinophilia of the blood and sputum. Bronchial casts containing *A. fumigatus* may be expectorated, precipitins to the fungus are commonly present in the blood, and skin tests with *Aspergillus* antigen cause both immediate and late reactions. The late reaction, which is elicited with an intradermal test solution, appears four hours after the test and is inhibited by corticosteroids. Bronchial challenge with *Aspergillus* antigen may produce positive immediate and late bronchial (asthmatic) reactions.

INVESTIGATIONS

A diagnosis of bronchial asthma is made chiefly on clinical grounds, and in the assessment of the wheezy patient it is essential to obtain a detailed history. This includes information about the frequency and severity of attacks, details of precipitating factors, history of allergy, smoking history, family history and the details of previous treatment. The severity of the asthma can be assessed by enquiring about the time lost from school and work, the frequency of nocturnal wheeze, and the frequency of use of bronchodilator aerosols and corticosteroids.

Chest radiograph. During an acute attack the chest radiograph shows hyperinflation of the lungs, and the diaphragm is low and flat. Asthma does not usually cause shadowing in the lung fields unless pneumonia or allergic bronchopulmonary aspergillosis are present. In children with severe chronic asthma there may be streaky shadows radiating from the hilum. A chest radiograph should be taken to exclude a pneumothorax which is an occasional complication of acute asthma. Pneumothorax, especially if shallow, may otherwise be overlooked because severe wheeze can mask the signs of air in the pleural space.

Sputum examination. Bacterial pathogens may be isolated from patients with acute asthma. Eosinophils are commonly present in large numbers but are rarely numerous in bronchitis.

Peripheral blood. Eosinophilia is common in both extrinsic and intrinsic asthma but the absolute count is usually less than 1000/mm^3

unless the asthma is a manifestation of pulmonary eosinophilia. Eosinophilia is not a feature of bronchitis. The haemoglobin, total white cell count and ESR are usually normal.

Pulmonary function tests. Measurement of FEV_1 and FVC and/or PEFR are essential. These tests indicate the severity of airways obstruction and are measured daily in hospital patients, and when possible should be measured in out-patients.

The FEV_1 and FEV_1/FVC ratio are both reduced when airways obstruction is present. During an acute attack the FEV_1 is often less than 1.0 litre and the FEV_1/FVC ratio is below 30 per cent. In most cases these levels improve within a few days of begining treatment and are a good indication of the patient's progress. The transfer factor is usually normal in asthma but is reduced in emphysema.

Reversibility studies. The degree of reversibility of the airways obstruction if assessed by measuring ventilatory function before and 30 minutes after bronchodilators. Drugs used in this assessment include aerosols of salbutamol, terbutaline or rimiterol. A 20 per cent rise in FEV_1 or PEFR suggests asthma; in chronic bronchitis and emphysema there is either no response or response of < 15 per cent.

Response to corticosteroids. In chronic asthma, assessment of ventilatory response to corticosteroids is imperative in the selection of patients for long-term corticosteroid therapy. When the clinical condition permits, baseline measurement of FEV_1 and/or PEFR are obtained while the patient is given a placebo for several days. Prednisolone, 20–40 mg daily, is then given for up to 3 weeks and FEV_1 and/or PEFR are recorded daily (Fig. 18). A 20 per cent increase during treatment with prednisolone indicates a significant response to corticosteroids.

This assessment can also be used to select an appropriate prednisolone treatment regimen. If there has been significant improvement after prednisolone, the placebo is re-introduced and measurements are continued for a further four days to determine the duration of remission. If the FEV_1 falls within 24 hours of stopping prednisolone it is probable that the patient will need daily treatment, but if the FEV_1 is maintained for several days it is possible that intermittent treatment will be effective (p. 124). Many patients previously managed by intermittent prednisolone therapy are now usually controlled satisfactorily with daily inhaled corticosteroids.

Blood gas analysis. This should be carried out in all patients with status asthmaticus. Hypoxaemia is frequently present and is often more severe than is suspected clinically. Knowledge of the P_aO_2 and P_aCO_2 allows correct selection of oxygen concentration. Usually the

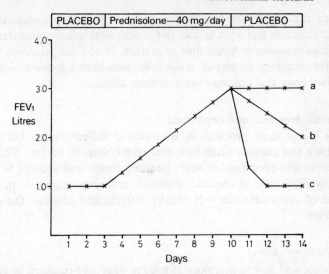

Fig. 18 Assessment of ventilatory response to corticosteroids. After stopping prednisolone the FEV_1 may be maintained (a); it may fall gradually over several days (b); or it may fall within 24 hours (c).

P_aCO_2 is low, but if it is raised it indicates serious hypoventilation and may determine the need for assisted ventilation.

Bronchial challenge. Bronchial hypersensitivity to a particular allergen may be assessed by measurement of ventilatory function before and after inhalation of the allergen. Bronchial challenge may precipitate severe asthma and is not done routinely.

Skin tests. There are numerous antigens available to test skin hypersensitivity. The prick test is the safest method and development of a weal and erythema at the test site after 15 minutes indicates a positive reaction. A positive skin test does not imply bronchial hypersensitivity. Positive results must be correlated with the patient's history and are of doubtful clinical significance if the patient denies that contact with the particular allergen causes asthma. Skin tests are most useful in confirming hypersensitivity to specific allergens which are suspected as being aetiologically significant from the history. Antihistamines, but not corticosteroids, can render the skin tests negative.

DIFFERENTIAL DIAGNOSIS

Acute bronchitis
Recurrent attacks of acute bronchitis are common in childhood and may be very difficult to differentiate from asthma. In recurrent bron-

chitis the attacks are usually precipitated by an upper respiratory tract infection and wheeze does not occur under other circumstances such as exposure to house dust or pollens. In addition, children who suffer recurrent attacks of acute bronchitis have a lower incidence of hay fever and eczema than asthmatic children.

Chronic bronchitis and emphysema

The commonest problem in diagnosis is differentiation between asthma and chronic bronchitis and emphysema in adults. Wheeze in a middle-aged smoker with morning cough and sputum is virtually diagnostic of chronic bronchitis and emphysema. A proper trial of corticosteroids will usually differentiate between the conditions.

Pulmonary oedema

Wheeze and severe dyspnoea of sudden onset are common in acute pulmonary oedema ('cardiac asthma'). This diagnosis must be considered if the patient is elderly and has noticed recent progressive deterioration in exercise tolerance. Widespread crepitations and cardiomegaly confirm the diagnosis. Usually there is evidence of an underlying cause of cardiac failure and the diagnosis can be confirmed by chest radiography and electrocardiography.

Pulmonary embolism

This causes sudden severe breathlessness but rarely causes wheeze or rhonchi.

TREATMENT

Treatment is based on the appropriate use of bronchodilators, corticosteroids and antibiotics. Avoidance of allergens and treatment with sodium cromoglycate may prevent asthma attacks due to allergy. Hyposensitisation is frequently helpful in pure grass pollen asthma.

The general principles of bronchodilator, corticosteroid and antibiotic therapy have been discussed in Chapter 6. The patient must always be taught how to use a bronchodilator inhaler properly and also warned that if he requires his inhaler more often than every three hours it is an indication that other treatment, usually with systemic corticosteroids, is necessary. Medical advice should be sought sooner rather than later.

Episodic asthma

A β_2 sympathomimetic inhaler is often sufficient to relieve a mild attack. Aminophylline i.v., 250 to 500 mg, may be necessary to relieve more severe wheeze, and if the attack persists, prednisolone, 20 to 40 mg daily, should be given until the attack remits and then rapidly tailed off. Patients requiring more than one such course are likely to require regular prophylactic cromoglycate or inhaled corticosteroids. Slow-release preparations of theophylline or aminophylline, given at bedtime or twice per 24 hours will sometimes prevent nocturnal wheeze or morning dipping. If an attack is precipitated by infection a five day course of ampicillin or tetracycline, 250 mg 6–8 hourly, should be given.

Status asthmaticus

Table 13 outlines the treatment of status asthmaticus. Oxygen is imperative and is given in high concentration, ⩾ 35 per cent. It is vital that the airway is kept clear by regular assisted coughing and physiotherapy, and adequate hydration makes the secretions less tenacious. *Sedation is dangerous and should be avoided*. Restlessness and agitation in acute asthma are due to hypoxaemia and must not be misinterpreted as psychological symptoms.

i.v. hydrocortisone in a dose of 1–2 g in the first 24 hours should be given and oral prednisolone started at the same time, 40 mg Stat and 10 mg 6 hourly. Potassium supplements should be given while such high doses of corticosteroids are maintained. After 24–36 hours hydrocortisone can be discontinued.

i.v. aminophylline is given as slow bolus injections, 250–500 mg 6 hourly, or as constant infusion, for 24–48 hours. Nebulised sal-

Table 13 Treatment of status asthmaticus

Oxygen	35%, ± humidification.
Maintain a clear airway	Assisted coughing, physiotherapy
Corticosteroids	Hydrocortisone I.V. 250 mg stat and 100 mg 2 hourly
	+
	Prednisolone 40 mg stat and 10 mg 6 hourly.
Bronchodilators	Aminophylline I.V. 0.25 to 0.5 g 6 hourly.
	and/or
	Nebulised β_2 sympathomimetic 4 hourly (see Table 7 for doses)
Antibiotics	Ampicillin 250 mg 6 hourly
	or
	Tetracycline 250 mg 6 hourly
Adequate hydration	
No sedation	

butamol (5 mg in 4 ml) or terbutaline (2.5–5 mg in 4 ml) or other β_2 sympathomimetic is given every 4–6 hours using flow rates of 8 l/min of oxygen to nebulise the solutions.

Antibiotics are usually given although some physicians will await the results of sputum culture if the patient is apyrexial and if infection has not been an obvious precipitant.

Exhaustion, confusion, progressive hypoxaemia, hypercapnia and a fall in pH are all serious signs. Assisted ventilation with sedation is sometimes indicated if the P_aO_2 is persistently less than 40 mmHg and the $P_a CO_2$ is above 50 mmHg. In practice, assisted ventilation is rarely necessary if other measures, particularly corticosteroids, are started early.

Chronic asthma

Regular treatment with bronchodilators may control the wheeze of chronic asthma, and cromoglycate and avoidance of allergens are helpful in cases with an allergic basis. Antibiotics are often given prophylactically at the onset of an upper respiratory infection in order to prevent acute attacks of asthma. Short courses of prednisolone may be necessary during acute attacks.

Long term corticosteroid therapy

Sometimes regular long-term treatment with corticosteroids is necessary and this decision is initially based on the severity of the asthma and thefrequency of acute attacks. Persistent daily wheeze and frequent absence from school or work, despite bronchodilator and cromoglycate therapy, are indications for long term treatment. Objective assessment should always be carried out to determine whether corticosteroids produce a significant increase in ventilatory levels and to aid selection of an appropriate regimen for long term treatment (p. 120).

Prednisolone dosage for daily treatment is usually 10 mg or less, and side effects are uncommon with this dose. Intermittent regimens include alternate day treatment, treatment on two consecutive days in four, and treatment on three consecutive days each week. The aim of long term treatment is to use the lowest dose which will control symptoms. The frequency of side effects such as hypercorticism, peripheral oedema and spontaneous fractures is lower with intermittent regimens than with daily treatment.

Patients on long term treatment should temporarily increase the dose of prednisolone as soon as they develop an acute attack and report to their doctor. All patients should carry a 'steroid' card giving relevant details which may be used in an emergency. Regular supervision of long term corticosteroid therapy is essential, and watch must be maintained for reactivation of tuberculosis and the development of diabetes mellitus.

Beclomethasone dipropionate or *betamethasone valerate* by inhaler, 400–800 µg daily, have enabled many patients to reduce gradually or discontinue oral corticosteroids. Many new asthmatics who previously would have needed systemic treatment with corticosteroids can now be managed on regular inhaled corticosteroid and p.r.n. inhaled bronchodilator, supplemented by oral theophyllines in some. Oropharyngeal thrush appears to be the only significant side-effect of inhaled corticosteroids, a marked contrast to the problems encountered with systemic steroids. During acute attacks patients on inhaled corticosteroids will need short, high-dose courses of prednisolone.

Corticotrophin (ACTH) is sometimes used in place of prednisolone in children with chronic asthma too young to use a pressurised inhaler since it causes less retardation of growth.

Avoidance of allergens

Avoidance of allergens is important in patients whose asthma is clearly allergic to origin. The following general measures may also be beneficial when there is a less obvious allergic basis. Avoidance of undue exposure to house dust is essential, particularly in the patient's bedroom. Furniture which collects dust should be kept to a minimum, curtains should be replaced by a roll-up blind and the patient's bed should be covered during the day. Lino or polished wood floors are preferable to carpets. The bedroom should be dusted daily with a damp cloth to avoid dust dispersal. Kapok or feather pillows should be replaced by a foam rubber pillow, woollen blankets by artificial fibre and the mattress should be turned daily. Regular vacuum cleaning of the mattress and blankets may reduce the number of mites. Similar measures are advisable for the rest of the house and soft toys. Allergenic pets should not be kept.

Patients with purely grass pollen asthma often benefit from hyposensitising injections given in two successive years in the early spring. Benefit from hyposensitisation to house dust mite has not been conclusively shown. Occasionally exclusion of milk products from the diet will produce dramatic improvement in childhood asthma.

Sodium cromoglycate (*Intal*)

This is used for prophylactic treatment and it is often effective in asthma which is precipitated by allergy or exercise. It is less effective in asthma which is not caused by known allergens and in such patients inhaled corticosteroids are preferable. Sodium cromoglycate probably acts on the mast cell and blocks the release of the pharmacological mediators which cause bronchial constriction.

Sodium cromoglycate is a white powder which is inhaled from a capsule using a special inhaler. Except in exercise induced asthma there is a latent period of 2 to 3 weeks before it is effective and it does not give symptomatic relief in acute attacks. The usual dose is one capsule qid, but after an interval a gradual reduction in dose may be possible. There are no serious side-effects but occasionally it causes coughing attacks due to bronchial irritation.

General measures

Asthma patients rarely require psychiatric treatment but they benefit greatly from the support of an understanding doctor. Regular attendance at a special asthma clinic also helps to provide a sense of security and to educate the patients and their relatives about the disease and its treatment. Hypnosis and acupuncture are of limited value and rarely provide lasting benefit.

FURTHER READING

British Medical Journal 1971 Therapeutic Conferences i:220
British Thoracic Association 1982 Death from asthma in two regions of England. British Medical Journal 285:1251
British Thoracic & Tuberculosis Association 1975 Inhaled corticosteroids compared with oral prednisone in patients starting long-term corticosteroid therapy for asthma. Lancet ii:469
British Thoracic & Tuberculosis Association 1976 A controlled trial of inhaled corticosteroids in patients receiving prednisone tablets for asthma. British Journal Diseases of the Chest 70:95
Clark T J H, Godfrey S 1977 Asthma. Chapman and Hall, London
Mygind N, Clark T J H 1980 Topical steroid treatment for asthma and rhinitis. Balliere Tindall, London
Rees H A, Millar J S, Donald K W 1968 A study of the clinical course and arterial blood gas tensions of patients in status asthmaticus. Quarterly Journal of Medicine 37:541
Rudd R M, Wedzicha J 1982 Asthma. Seminar. Update Supplement. Update Publications Ltd, London

13

Chronic bronchitis and emphysema

DEFINITIONS

Chronic bronchitis

The Medical Research Council defines chronic bronchitis as a disease characterized by cough productive of sputum on most days during at least three consecutive months for more than two successive years. This definition assumes that diseases such as bronchiectasis and tuberculosis, which also cause chronic cough and sputum, have been excluded. The sputum may be mucoid or mucopurulent. The main functional abnormality is persistent generalized airways obstruction which results in wheeze and breathlessness.

Emphysema and bronchial asthma also cause generalized airways obstruction and this may lead to difficulty in diagnosis which is accentuated by the fact that about most patients with chronic bronchitis also have emphysema.

Emphysema.

Emphysema is defined in pathological terms as a condition characterized by increase beyond the normal in the size of the air spaces distal to the terminal bronchiole. Emphysema may occur as the only abnormality (*primary emphysema*) but more commonly it occurs in association with chronic bronchitis. In both types of emphysema there is airways obstruction. Severe breathlessness is the main symptom of emphysema. In emphysema associated with chronic bronchitis the clinical features include cough, sputum, wheeze and breathlessness.

In bronchial asthma the airways obstruction changes in severity over short periods of time either spontaneously or as a result of treatment. This causes recurrent paroxysmal attacks of wheeze and breathlessness. Usually asthma can be differentiated from chronic bronchitis by its episodic nature, but diagnosis may be difficult in chronic asthma where there is persistent airways obstruction. Persistent cough, and sputum are not dominant symptoms of asthma

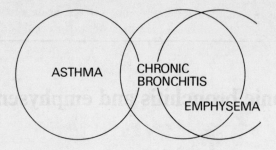

Fig. 19 The relationship between asthma, chronic bronchitis and emphysema.

although occasionally asthma and chronic bronchitis coexist. Asthma is rarely complicated by emphysema.

Since airways obstruction is the functional disorder common to these diseases they are sometimes given the name 'chronic obstructive lung disease'. Most authorities consider that this term is confusing and should not be used. It is preferable to differentiate between the diseases that cause airways obstruction. Figure 19 illustrates the spectrum of airways obstruction and the relationship between asthma, chronic bronchitis and emphysema.

CHRONIC BRONCHITIS

Epidemiology

The prevalence of chronic bronchitis varies considerably from country and is highest in Britain where 10 to 15 per cent of middle-aged men are affected. The prevalence increases with age, cigarette consumption and atmospheric pollution. Chronic bronchitis is more common in urban than rural dwellers and is more prevalent in the lower socio-economic groups. Men are affected five times more frequently than women and there is a higher prevalence in occupations such as coal mining. In Britain 35 million working days are lost each year through illness from bronchitis. The mortality rate from chronic bronchitis is 80 per 100 000 and is highest during the winter months.

Aetiology

The major aetiological factors are tobacco smoking, atmospheric pollution and infection. Smoking and atmospheric pollution cause chronic bronchial irritation and predispose to recurrent acute respiratory infections. After many years these factors produce the functional and structural changes of chronic bronchitis. Occupation, socio-economic status and heredity may also play an aetiological role, but the significance of these factors is difficult to evaluate because they may be related to smoking habits and atmospheric pollution.

Smoking

Epidemiological studies have shown a causal relationship between tobacco smoking and chronic bronchitis. Non smokers rarely develop chronic bronchitis and among smokers, morbidity and mortality are closely related to the number of cigarettes smoked. A survey of British doctors showed that the death rate from chronic bronchitis among those who smoked 25 or more cigarettes daily was over 20 times higher than in non-smokers. Subsequently there was a fall in death rates among doctors who had stopped smoking for more than five years. There is also reduction in cough and sputum after smoking is stopped. Cigar and pipe smoking predispose to chronic bronchitis but are less harmful than cigarette smoking. The immediate effect of smoking a cigarette is a sudden increase in airways resistance. This bronchoconstriction is probably mediated through the vagus nerve since it is inhibited by atropine. Constant heavy smoking for many years causes hypertrophy of the mucous glands of the bronchial tree, increase in the number of goblet cells and hypersecretion of mucus. Smoking also interferes with the action of the bronchial cilia which contributes to the accumulation of mucus in the bronchial tree.

Atmospheric pollution

Pollution of the atmosphere by industrial and domestic smoke plays a less important aetiological role than cigarette smoking. There is, however, a correlation between atmospheric pollution and the prevalence of chronic bronchitis. Atmospheric pollution accounts for the higher morbidity and mortality rates in urban than in rural dwellers. Sulphur dioxide is one of the components of polluted air and causes bronchial irritation and increased airways resistance. Atmospheric pollution may account partly for the higher incidence of chronic bronchitis in the lower socio-economic groups and in certain occupations.

Infection

The role of infection in initiating chronic bronchitis is not clear, but once the disease is established recurrent bronchial infections are common and cause progressive bronchial damage and emphysema. Exacerbations of chronic bronchitis are mainly caused by *H. influenzae* or *Str. pneumoniae*. Specific precipitins to *H. influenzae* can be

demonstrated in some patients and confirm the aetiological importance of this organism. Exacerbations of chronic bronchitis sometimes follow a cold or other upper respiratory tract infection.
Exacerbations are common during the winter months and this may
be related to the winter prevalence of upper respiratory infections,
overcrowding and increased atmospheric pollution. Changes in temperature and humidity may aggravate symptoms but probably do
not initiate acute exacerbations.

Pathogenesis, pathology and functional abnormality

Mucous gland hypertrophy. The main pathological finding in
chronic bronchitis is hypertrophy of the mucous glands of the bronchial tree. (Fig. 20). This is the result of chronic irritation by
cigarette smoke and atmospheric pollution. Reid showed that the
degree of mucous gland hypertrophy may be estimated by compar-
ing the gland thickness with the thickness of the bronchial wall. The
bronchial wall thickness is measured from the epithelium to the cartilage layer; the gland thickness is measured at the same point. The
gland to wall ratio is known as the Reid Index. Increase in the Reid
Index is the best criterion for the pathological diagnosis of chronic
bronchitis.

Goblet cells. The number of goblet cells in the bronchial epithelium is increased, particularly in the small airways.

Hypersecretion of mucus. Mucous gland hypertrophy and increase
in the number of goblet cells result in hypersecretion of mucus and
the characteristic symptoms of chronic cough and sputum. The

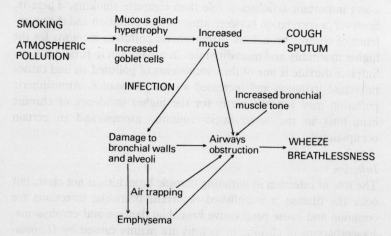

Fig. 20 Pathogenesis of chronic bronchitis.

mucous glands mainly contribute to the increased sputum volume; goblet cell hypersecretion is mainly responsible for blockage of peripheral airways. The increased secretions line the bronchial tree and are one of the factors which cause airways obstruction and wheeze. The accumulated secretions provide a good culture medium for bacteria.

Infection of bronchioles and alveoli. Hypersecretion predisposes to lower respiratory tract infections. The bronchial walls are infiltrated with inflammatory cells and there is dilatation of bronchial capillaries and lymphatics. Recurrent infections cause irreversible fibrosis and destruction of the walls of the small bronchi, bronchioles and alveoli.

Emphysema. In most patients with chronic bronchitis emphysema is present. It results from destruction of the walls of the bronchioles and alveoli by repeated infections and from distension of alveoli by air trapping. Air trapping is caused by loss of pulmonary elastic recoil and by premature closure of weakened peripheral airways during expiration. The emphysema may involve the alveoli within the centre of the acinus (centriacinar emphysema) or the alveoli throughout the acinus (panacinar emphysema).

Airways obstruction. This is the main functional abnormality and is caused by any or all of the following factors: mucus lining the bronchial tree, narrowing of the bronchial walls by inflammation, increased bronchial muscle tone, narrowing of the peripheral airways by fibrosis, air trapping and emphysema. Early in the disease the airways obstruction is intermittent and may only be present when acute infection causes increased secretions and inflammatory narrowing of the bronchi. Later, the airways obstruction is persistent although it may be temporarily relieved by bronchodilators. Corticosteroids do not produce significant bronchodilation in chronic bronchitis.

The airways obstruction is most easily demonstrated by ventilatory function tests which show an obstructive defect. Airways obstruction produces ventilation-perfusion inequality which results in hypoxaemia, although initially this is present only during exacerbations. Severe airways obstruction causes alveolar hypoventilation and the $P_a CO_2$ rises especially during exacerbations. In patients with hypercapnia the respiratory centre no longer responds to carbon dioxide and hypoxaemia becomes the main stimulus to respiration. Treatment with high concentrations of oxygen removes this stimulus and increases the degree of hypoventilation, resulting in a further rise in $P_a CO_2$. In severe ventilatory failure, hypercapnia causes respiratory acidosis with a fall in pH and a compensatory rise in plasma bicarbonate. Hypoxaemia and hypercapnia affect cerebral and cardiovascular function.

Severe airways obstruction causes hyperinflation of the lungs which is shown by increase in RV and RV/TLC ratio. The transfer factor is normal in chronic bronchitis.

Cor pulmonale. Patients with severe chronic bronchitis frequently develop right ventricular failure although the precise reason for this is not clear. During exacerbations of infection, hypoxaemia may cause pulmonary vasoconstriction and temporary pulmonary hypertension.

Clinical features

Cough and sputum are the predominant early symptoms of chronic bronchitis, but in the later stages *wheeze* and *breathlessness* become marked. The following description illustrates the characteristic presentation and course of the disease.

Usually the patient is a man who has smoked heavily for many years and symptoms begin insidiously after the age of 40. Cough and sputum on waking are the first symptoms but initially they are so slight that they are regarded as 'only a smoker's cough'. At first the sputum is mucoid and only becomes purulent during winter attacks of acute bronchitis. If the patient continues to smoke there is slow but progressive worsening of symptoms. Sputum is more copious and the early morning coughing attacks are now accompanied by wheeze which persists until the patient has expectorated the secretions which have accumulated over-night. Unlike the patient with asthma, sleep is not usually disturbed by attacks of nocturnal wheeze. The patient notices decrease in exercise tolerance, and running for a bus or climbing stairs causes wheeze and breathlessness. Attacks of winter bronchitis become more frequent and the patient takes longer to recover.

In the later stages the patient is very disabled. His chest is never completely free of secretions and attacks of coughing are precipitated by exertion, smoke, fog and sudden changes in temperature. The sputum may now be persistently mucopurulent. Wheeze and breathlessness are precipitated by minimal exertion and sometimes even shaving becomes laborious. The patient can no longer work and may only venture outside to visit the doctor.

Physical examination. Scattered inspiratory and expiratory rhonchi are the main finding. The rhonchi are loudest during expiration which is usually prolonged. In mild cases rhonchi may only be heard on forced expiration and this is a useful manoeuvre if bronchitis is suspected. The rhonchi are variable in pitch but are often low pitched and loudest over the lower lobes: they cannot be differen- tiated from rhonchi due to asthma. Chronic bronchitis does not cause finger clubbing.

The other signs depend on the severity of the airways obstruction, the degree of hypoxaemia and hypercapnia, and the presence of emphysema and cor pulmonale:

Severe airways obstruction. Dyspnoea on minimal exertion, use of the accessory muscles of respiration, central cyanosis, audible wheeze and inspiratory indrawing of the lower intercostal spaces indicate severe airways obstruction. The patient often breathes through partly closed lips. This is called 'pursed lip breathing' and results from an attempt to maintain a pressure gradient in the bron- chial tree and so minimize air trapping. Hyperinflation is common and on percussion the upper level of liver dullness is below the 6th rib in the right midclavicular line. Terminally these patients develop right ventricular failure and because of the oedema and cyanosis they are sometimes colloquially referred to as 'blue and bloated'.

Hypoxaemia and hypercapnia. These cause mental confusion and impaired level of consciousness. Coma, coarse muscle twitching, flapping tremor, warm extremities, collapsing pulse and papilloe- dema are signs of hypercapnia (p. 145).

Emphysema. Emphysema may cause a barrel shaped chest with increase in the anteroposterior diameter, marked limitation of chest expansion, hyperresonant percussion note with decrease of liver dullness, faint heart sounds and decreased intensity of the breath sounds. These signs are suggestive of emphysema but are not diag- nostic. Other signs which have been attributed to emphysema are even less reliable. In fact, the clinical diagnosis of emphysema is often very difficult. Hyperinflation with loss of liver dullness is prob- ably the most reliable sign although it may also occur in chronic bronchitis without emphysema and in acute asthma.

Cor pulmonale. Raised jugular venous pressure, hepatomegaly and ankle oedema indicate right ventricular failure. These signs must be elicited carefully because jugular venous distension occurs normally during forced expiration while a palpable liver may be due to depression of the diaphragm from hyperinflation.

Investigations

Chest radiograph. The chest radiograph is usually normal in chronic bronchitis. There may be hyperinflation with a low flat dia- phragm, although this is more common in patients with emphysema. The most reliable signs of emphysema are attenuation and narrowing of the peripheral vessels of the lungs and a large retorsternal translucent zone. These findings are only obvious in severe emphysema and in the majority of cases the diagnosis cannot be made with confidence from the chest radiograph. Enlargement of the pulmonary arteries may indicate pulmonary hypertension, but this finding is uncommon.

Peripheral blood. This is usually normal. Leucocytosis and elevation of the ESR are not consistent findings during an exacerbation of chronic bronchitis. Polycythaemia occasionally occurs in longstanding chronic bronchitis and emphysema.

Sputum examination. Pus cells are often present and during exacerbations *H. influenzae* or *Str. pneumoniae* are often isolated.

Pulmonary function tests. Reduction of FEV_1 and an FEV_1/FVC ratio of less than 65 per cent indicate airways obstruction. In patients with severe chronic bronchitis the FEV_1 is less than 1 l and $FEV_1/FVC < 30$ per cent. Improvement of ventilatory function after a bronchodilator is more common in chronic bronchitis than emphysema. Corticosteroids do not produce $\geqslant 20$ per cent improvement in ventilatory levels in chronic bronchitis or emphysema: if there is improvement, it is probable that the patient has asthma. In both chronic bronchitis and emphysema there is increase in RV and RV/TLC ratio. In emphysema the TLC is also increased. In chronic bronchitis without emphysema the transfer factor is normal.

Blood gas analysis. Initially blood gas analysis is normal. As the disease progresses, hypoxaemia, hypercapnia and respiratory acidosis may occur during exacerbations. In a typical case the results of blood gas analysis might show $P_a CO_2$ 70 mmHg and pH 7.3. Chronic hypoxaemia and hypercapnia do not usually occur until the FEV_1 is persistently below 1 l.

Differential diagnosis

Emphysema and asthma.

The main problem in diagnosis is the differentiation between chronic bronchitis, emphysema and asthma. Many patients with chronic bronchitis also have emphysema but unless the emphysema is severe it is masked by the features of bronchitis. Sometimes emphysema is the dominant or only abnormality and gives rise to characteristic features (p. 140). Table 14 contrasts 'pure examples' of these three conditions.

Typically in asthma there is a history of paroxysmal attacks of wheeze beginning in childhood. The diagnosis is more difficult if symptoms first appear in adult life. In these cases factors which favour a diagnosis of asthma include a family history of the disease, attacks of nocturnal wheezing, freedom from chronic cough and sputum and absence of a history of cigarette smoking. Occasionally patients have features of both chronic bronchitis and asthma.

Table 14 Differentiation between chronic bronchitis, emphysema and asthma

	Chronic bronchitis	Emphysema	Bronchial asthma
Age of onset	>40 years	Often in childhood	.
Family history of asthma	Uncommon	Uncommon	Common
Personal history of allergy	Uncommon	Uncommon	Common
Smoking history	Smoker	Smoker	Non-smoker
Early symptoms	Persistent morning cough and sputum	Breathlessness	Paroxysms of wheeze
Infective episodes	Common	Occasional	Variable
Exercise tolerance	Often reduced	Poor	Often normal in remissions
General cyanosis	Common in late stages ('blue and bloated')	Absent ('pink puffer')	Absent except during severe attack
Wheeze, rhonchi	Present	Often inaudible	Present during attack
Chest radiograph	Often normal	Pruning of peripheral vessels	Hyperinflation
Blood eosinophilia	Absent	Absent	Often present
Skin tests	Negative	Negative	Positive
FEV$_1$ ⎫ FEV$_1$/FVC ⎭	Low	Very low	Low during attack Responds to corticosteroids
P$_a$O$_2$	Normal or low	Normal or slightly reduced	Low during acute attack
P$_a$CO$_2$	Normal or raised	Normal or low	Normal or low
Transfer factor	Normal	Low	Normal
Right ventricular failure	Relatively early	Late	Absent
Prognosis	Poor	Very poor	Good

Bronchial carcinoma
Bronchial carcinoma and chronic bronchitis frequently coexist since smoking is the common aetiological factor. Carcinoma should be suspected if haemoptysis, finger clubbing, pneumonia or a radiographic abnormality occur in any patient with chronic bronchitis.

Bronchiectasis
The history of cough and sputum usually dates from childhood, wheeze is not usually a dominant symptom and the sputum is more copious.

Tuberculosis
This must be considered in any patient with chronic cough but can be dismissed if the chest radiograph is normal.

Treatment
Long term treatment
The most important measure is to convince the patient to stop smoking. He should be told that his symptoms are due to smoking and encouraged to seek the support of his family and friends in an attempt to give up the habit. Anti-smoking clinics have met with limited success. In the later stages of the disease the medical social worker and community services such as 'meals on wheels' can do much to support the patient.

Bronchodilators. These are given if they produce symptomatic and/or objective improvement, and the principles of treatment and the different preparations are discussed on page 60. Corticosteroids are not indicated unless objective assessment shows that they produce 20 per cent increase in ventilatory levels (p. 120).

Antibiotics. Tetracycline, 250 mg qds, or ampicillin 250 mg tds, are the antibiotics of choice and rarely cause side effects. The patient with frequent exacerbations of infection should be given a home supply with instructions to start treatment as soon as an exacerbation begins. Sulfametopyrazine given once a week as a prophylactic in winter can halve the number of exacerbations. Preventive chemotherapy has not been shown to prevent functional deterioration.

Mucolytic agents. These are ineffective in aiding expectoration except in patients with scanty mucoid sputum and minimal dyspnoea.

Diuretics and digitalis. Thiazides, and later, frusemide, will usually control oedema due to cor pulmonale. Digitalis is indicated if there is atrial fibrillation or severe cardiac failure.

Domiciliary oxygen. In the later stages of the disease an oxygen cylinder in the home provides considerable symptomatic relief, and portable oxygen increases the patient's mobility. The oxygen must be given by 24 or 28 per cent Ventimask, and the patient and his relatives must be warned about the inflammable nature or oxygen. Domiciliary oxygen for ten or more hours per day can improve and prolong life.

Treatment of acute exacerbations
Table 15 shows a plan of treatment for acute exacerbations of chronic bronchitis.

Oxygen. If hypoxaemia is present, or is suspected, 24 per cent oxygen is given by Ventimask. If this does not cause drowsiness or a rise in P_a CO_2 the concentration may be increased to 28 per cent. Blood gas analysis is essential during a severe exacerbation.

Maintain a clear airway. This is of vital importance and the patient must be told that it is imperative for him to cough up phlegm. Regular assisted coughing should be supervised by the nursing staff and physiotherapist and it may be necessary to do this hourly. Adequate fluids keep the secretions loose and assist expectoration. Early and constant attention to the airway, with the aid of nikethamide or doxapram, will often avoid the necessity for bronchoscopy and assisted ventilation.

Bronchodilators. Nebulised bronchodilator will alleviate acute airways obstruction and may be repeated every four hours. This treatment facilitates expectoration and should be followed by assisted coughing. Many patients find I.V. aminophylline helpful also (250–500 mg I.V. slowly every six hours or as constant infusion, 5 mg/kg loading dose over 20 minutes followed by 1 mg/kg/hour). As recovery takes place an ordinary pressurised inhaler and tablet theophylline should suffice.

Antibiotics. The majority of exacerbations are due to infection and antibiotics are given routinely. Tetracycline or ampicillin, 250 mg 6 or 8 hourly, are usually effective. A combination of trimethoprim

Table 15   Treatment of an acute exacerbation of chronic bronchitis

Oxygen	24 to 28% by Ventimask
Maintain a clear airway	Assisted coughing, physiotherapy, respiratory stimulant
Bronchodilators	Nebulised bronchodilator and/or i.v. aminophylline
	Later: bronchodilator inhaler ± oral theophylline
Antibiotics	Ampicillin 250 mg 8 hourly or Tetracycline 250 mg 6 hourly
Adequate hydration	Orally or 5% dextrose i.v.
No sedation	

and sulphamethoxaole (co-trimoxazole) is also used to treat acute exacerbations. Decrease in sputum purulence indicates response to treatment. Antibiotics are given for a week.

In the majority of cases the acute exacerbation resolves with these measures. Barbiturates and opiates must not be given because of the risk of causing respiratory depression. Occasionally assisted ventilation is necessary if, despite intensive treatment, there is persistent hypoxaemia with P_a O_2 less than 40 mmHg and a progressive rise in P_a CO_2 with pH below 7.25 (p. 148). It is sometimes difficult to justify assisted ventilation in a patient who has been severely incapacitated by breathlessness for many years before the exacerbation.

Prognosis

If the patient continues to smoke, chronic bronchitis is a slowly progressive disease and there is gradual increase in cough and sputum, and deterioration in respiratory function. Acute exacerbations occur with increasing frequency. Death is uncommon before the age of 50 but thereafter the mortality rises progressively. Chronic ventilatory failure and persistent cor pulmonale are bad prognostic signs and the patient rarely survives more than two years. The prevention of chronic bronchitis is discussed in the chapter on bronchial carcinoma.

EMPHYSEMA

There are two clinically important types of emphysema:

Emphysema associated with chronic bronchitis

Primary or idiopathic emphysema

Both cause airways obstruction and often severe respiratory disability.

Other types of emphysema are relatively unimportant because they do not usually give rise to severe symptoms. These include emphysema due to ageing of the lung, emphysema associated with coal miners' pneumoconiosis and compensatory emphysema due to overinflation of the lung after resection or collapse. A rare form of unilateral emphysema involving the whole lung may result from bronchitis and bronchial obstruction which interferes with lung development in childhood (Macleod's syndrome).

The following discussion applies only to emphysema associated with chronic bronchitis and primary emphysema.

Prevalence, aetiology and pathogenesis

Emphysema associated with chronic bronchitis is much commoner than primary emphysema. In Britain primary emphysema accounts for less than 10 per cent of all cases of emphysema. The proportion of patients with primary emphysema is higher in countries where chronic bronchitis is less prevalent.

Emphysema associated with chronic bronchitis is the result of recurrent infections which damage the walls of the bronchioles and alveoli. The peripheral airways lose the support of their alveolar attachments, and this creates a valve like effect during expiration, so that there is premature closure of the airways and air trapping. The increase in intrapulmonary pressure may cause expiratory collapse of the larger airways and trachea. The cause of primary emphysema is not known. The main abnormality is loss of pulmonary elastic recoil.

Deficiency of the enzyme α 1-antitrypsin is an inherited defect carried by an autosomal recessive gene. This enzyme normally circulates in the blood and is a potent inhibitor of proteolytic enzymes. It may protect the lung from the action of proteolytic enzymes, and it has been suggested that deficiency of α 1-antitrypsin allows bacterial enzymes to damage the lung parenchyma. The main features of this condition are a family history of emphysema, onset of exertional dyspnoea before the fifth decade, severe airways obstruction and pancinar emphysema mainly involving the lower lobes. Cigarette smoking hastens the onset of emphysema in persons with α 1-antitrypsin deficiency.

Pathology and functional abnormality

Emphysema associated with chronic bronchitis involves the centre of the acinus around the respiratory bronchiole—*centriacinar emphysema* (syn. centrilobular emphysema), the whole of the acinus—*panacinar emphysema* (syn. panlobular emphysema), or is distributed irregularly throughout the acinus. Commonly the emphysema is widespread throughout the lung.

In primary emphysema the lesions are predominantly panacinar. The bronchial tree is normal and does not show the characteristic mucous gland hypertrophy of chronic bronchitis. Gross emphysema of either type is associated with irreversible airways obstruction with decrease in FEV_1 and FEV_1/FVC ratio. Emphysema produces marked hyperinflation and the TLC, FRC, RV/TLC ratio are greatly increased. The transfer factor is decreased as a result of loss of surface for gas exchange. Pulmonary perfusion is reduced in emphysema and lung scans show gross irregular perfusion defects affecting most of the lung.

Emphysema produces ventilation-perfusion imbalance, but compensatory hyperventilation keeps the P_aCO_2 relatively normal if there is little or no associated chronic bronchitis. The hyperventilation and the absence of central cyanosis has led to use of the term 'pink puffer' to describe patients in whom emphysema is the dominant abnormality. The P_aCO_2 is normal or low as a result of hyper-ventilation. As the disease progresses P_aO_2 falls, P_aCO_2 rises and cor pulmonale supervenes.

Clinical and radiographic features

Progressive breathlessness is the predominant symptom of emphysema. Cough and sputum are minimal or absent in patients without chronic bronchitis.

Physical examination. Extreme dyspnoea without cyanosis, prolonged expiration and soft breath sounds, often with no rhonchi, are typical findings. A barrel shaped chest, limitation of chest expansion, hyperresonant percussion note with loss of liver dullness and decreased intensity of the breath sounds are suggestive of emphysema but are not diagnostic.

The *chest radiograph* shows hyperinflation, a narrow mediastinum, small heart and loss of the peripheral vascular markings. The finding is best seen on whole lung tomograms.

Treatment and course

There is no specific treatment. Bronchodilators are sometimes appreciated, often increasing FVC more than FEV_1. Corticosteroids are ineffective. Respiratory infections should be treated promptly with antibiotics. The patient must be persuaded to stop smoking and if obese must lose weight. After many years of increasing breathlessness the patient finally develops ventilatory failure and right ventricular failure. These complications occur later in patients with primary emphysema than in those with chronic bronchitis and emphysema.

EMPHYSEMATOUS BULLAE

Emphysema from any cause may give rise to bullae. A bulla is defined as an emphysematous space greater than 1 cm in diameter. Rupture of a bulla causes pneumothorax (p. 236). Occasionally bullae are extremely large and are recognized in the chest radiograph as an area of increased translucency which does not contain lung markings. A thin line marks the wall of the bulla. Very large bullae cause breathlessness, but since they are usually associated with generalized emphysema and often chronic bronchitis, it is difficult to determine their contribution to the patient's symptoms. Occasionally resection of a single very large bulla is indicated if it is causing compression of healthy lung tissue.

FURTHER READING

Bates D V, Macklem P T, Christie R V 1971 Respiratory function in disease. Saunders, Philadelphia

Crofton J, Douglas A 1981 Respiratory diseases. Blackwell, Oxford

Davies D, Darke C S 1978 Sulphametopyrazine prophylaxis in chronic bronchitis. British Journal Diseases of the Chest 72:231

Fletcher C, Peto R, Tinker C, Speizer F E 1976 The natural history of chronic bronchitis and emphysema. An eight year study of early chronic obstructive lung disease in working men in London. Oxford University Press, Oxford

Hutchison D C S, Cook P J L, Barter C E, Harris H, Hugh-Jones P 1971 Pulmonary emphysema and α 1-antitrypsin deficiency. British Medical Journal i:689

Lambert P M, Reid D D 1970 Smoking, air pollution and bronchitis in Britain. Lancet i:853

Lancet 1965 Medical Research Council: Definition and classification of chronic bronchitis for clinical and epidemiological purposes. i:775

Mackay A D 1980 Amoxycillin vs ampicillin in treatment of exacerbations of chronic bronchitis. British Journal of Diseases of the Chest 74:379

May J R 1972 The chemotherapy of chronic bronchitis and allied disorders. English Universities Press, London

Reid Lynne 1967 The pathology of emphysema. Lloyd-Luke, London.

Royal College of Physicians 1977 Smoking or health. Pitman, London.

Royal College of Physicians 1981 Disabling chest disease: prevention and care. Journal of the Royal College of Physicians of London 15:69

14

Respiratory failure

DEFINITION

The main function of the respiratory system is to achieve adequate gas exchange between the blood and the air, so that arterial blood gas tensions of oxygen and carbon dioxide remain normal. Respiratory failure is present when the P_aO_2 is below 60 mmHg or the P_aCO_2 is above 49 mmHg in a person at rest, breathing air at sea level. These arbitrary values are useful levels on which to base the definition of respiratory failure. This definition does not take into account patients with incipient respiratory failure in whom blood gases are normal at rest but become abnormal on exercise. Respiratory failure may be acute or chronic.

CLASSIFICATION

There are two types of respiratory failure:
1. *Hypoxaemia with a normal or low P_aCO_2.*
2. *Hypoxaemia with a raised P_aCO_2.* This is often called *ventilatory failure* because elevation of the P_aCO_2 can only occur as the result of alveolar hypoventilation.

AETIOLOGY AND FUNCTIONAL ABNORMALITY

1. *Hypoxaemia with a normal or low P_aCO_2*

   Ventilation-perfusion imbalance This is the main mechanism responsible for this type of respiratory failure. If some alveoli receive too little ventilation in proportion to perfusion (low $\dot{V}A/\dot{Q}$) there is a fall in P_aO_2 and a rise in P_aCO_2 in the blood leaving these alveoli. In effect, blood is shunted past the alveoli without adequate gas exchange taking place (*venous admixture effect*). Any rise in P_aCO_2 of the mixed arterial blood will stimulate the respiratory centre and cause increased ventilation of other alveoli. This rapidly compensates for the rise in P_aCO_2 because the excretion of carbon dioxide is directly related to alveolar ventilation and the carbon dioxide dissociation curve is linear. However, hyperventilation will not compensate for hypoxaemia because blood leaving normally ventilated alveoli almost fully saturated with oxygen. Any increase in alveolar oxygen tension due to hyperventilation will not significantly increase the oxygen content of the blood because of the sigmoid shape of the oxygen dissociation curve.

For these reasons the overall effect of reduction in ventilation-perfusion ratio is a fall in P_aO_2 with maintenance of a normal P_aCO_2. Compensatory hyperventilation may even reduce the P_aCO_2 to such low levels that the pH rises causing *respiratory alkalosis*. The kidneys compensate by increased excretion of HCO'_3 and the plasma HCO'_3 falls.

Reduction in ventilation-perfusion ratio is the commonest cause of hypoxaemia. Hypoxaemia with a normal or low P_aCO_2 is always due to disease of the lung itself, and common examples include *asthma, pneumonia, pulmonary fibrosis, pulmonary oedema* and *pulmonary collapse*. Reduction in ventilation-perfusion ratio also contributes to the hypoxaemia of chronic bronchitis and emphysema.

Impaired gas transfer. Allergic alveolitis and *fibrosing alveolitis* may cause hypoxaemia with a normal or low P_aCO_2. These diseases involve the alveolar capillary membrane and may interfere with gas transfer across the membrane. However, the hypoxaemia is chiefly due to ventilation-perfusion imbalance.

2. Hypoxaemia with a raised P_aCO_2: ventilatory failure

Alveolar hypoventilation. The P_aCO_2 is the best index of the adequacy of alveolar ventilation, and it rises only if there is generalized alveolar hypoventilation. Alveolar ventilation may fall if the tidal volume or respiratory rate are reduced. This causes a rise in P_aCO_2 and a fall in P_aO_2. Because of the reciprocal relationship between the partial pressures of the two gases, the P_aCO_2 cannot rise above 90 mmHg while the patient is breathing air, without the P_aO_2 falling to near-lethal levels.

Alveolar hypoventilation is the main cause of hypoxaemia with a raised P_aCO_2. This type of respiratory failure may be caused by disorders which interfere with the respiratory pathway at any of the following sites: brain, spinal cord, intercostal nerves, neuromuscular junction, respiratory muscles, chest wall, airways and lungs (Fig. 21). The commonest cause of ventilatory failure is chronic bronchitis. In acute asthma, hyperventilation of adequately perfused alveoli usually prevents a rise in P_aCO_2. Hypercapnia may develop in severe status asthmaticus and indicates serious alveolar hypoventilation.

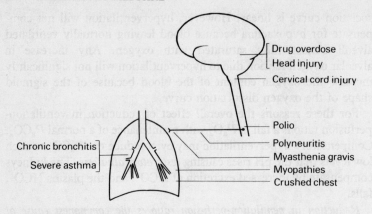

Fig. 21 Causes of ventilatory failure.

Ventilation-perfusion imbalance. Reduction in ventilation-perfusion ratio contributes to the hypoxaemia and hypercapnia of severe chronic bronchitis.

Elevation of P_aCO_2 causes a fall in pH and *respiratory acidosis*. If hypercapnia persists the kidneys conpensate for respiratory acidosis by excretion of H^+ and reabsorption of HCO'_3 so that the plasma HCO'_3 rises. Figure 22 summarizes the acid-base changes in respiratory acidosis and respiratory alkalosis. In patients with hypercapnia the normal sensitivity of the respiratory centre to carbon dioxide is reduced and hypoxaemia becomes the main stimulus to respiration. Treatment with high concentrations of oxygen corrects the

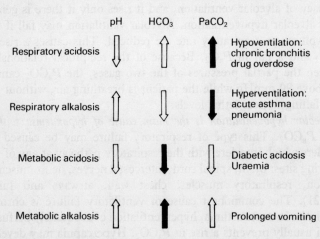

Fig. 22 Acid-base disturbance. The heavier arrows indicate the primary abnormality.

hypoxaemia but at the same time removes the stimulus to respiration so that ventilation is further reduced and P_aCO_2 rises to higher levels.

CLINICAL FEATURES

Respiratory failure may be *acute*, e.g. status asthmaticus, exacerbations of chronic bronchitis/emphysema or *chronic*, e.g. fibrosing alveolitis, late stages of chronic bronchitis/emphysema.

Breathlessness is not synonymous with respiratory failure. Many breathless patients have normal blood gases while some patients with severe hypoxaemia and hypercapnia are not breathless, e.g. drug overdose.

Respiratory arrest. Sometimes the first sign of respiratory failure is complete cessation of spontaneous respiration.

Central cyanosis. This is a reliable sign of respiratory failure, but it is a *late sign* and is only detected when the arterial oxygen saturation is below 80 per cent, at which stage the P_aO_2 is less than 50 mmHg.

Hypoxaemia. Hypoxaemia impairs cerebral function and causes restlessness, agitation and confusion. The heart responds to hypoxaemia by increase in heart rate and cardiac output, and if hypoxaemia is chronic, pulmonary hypertension and cor pulmonale may develop. Chronic hypoxaemia may cause polycythaemia. Severe hypoxaemia causes cardiac arrhythmias, renal failure and hepatic necrosis. Cellular damage occurs when the P_aO_2 falls below 20 mmHg. A serious consequence of severe hypoxaemia is accumulation of lactic acid and *metabolic acidosis* due to anaerobic tissue metabolism. The effects of hypoxaemia are more serious than the effects of hypercapnia.

Hypercapnia. Headache, confusion, drowsiness, coarse muscle twitching, flapping tremor, extensor plantar responses, coma and papilloedema are features of hypercapnia. Drowsiness and confusion are common when the P_aCO_2 is above 80 mmHg. Increasing drowsiness in patients with respiratory failure is usually due to increasing hypercapnia from excessive oxygen or sedation. Hypercapnia also causes peripheral vasodilatation resulting in sweating, warm extremities and collapsing pulse.

DIAGNOSIS

Blood gas analysis is essential for the diagnosis of respiratory failure because central cyanosis is a late sign, while the signs of hypoxaemia and hypercapnia are non-specific and correlate poorly with the severity of the respiratory failure. Respiratory failure should always be suspected in status asthmaticus, acute exacerbations of chronic bronchitis and severe pneumonia. Blood gas analysis is often carried out in these disorders to determine the adequacy of respiratory function and to enable correct choice of oxygen therapy. Repeated estimations may be necessary to monitor progress.

In the interpretation of the results of blood gas analysis it is important to know the concentration of oxygen the patient was breathing when the sample of blood was taken.

DIFFERENTIAL DIAGNOSIS

Cyanotic heart disease
Central cyanosis due to respiratory failure disappears within a minute if the patient is given 30 per cent oxygen. Persistent cyanosis while breathing oxygen indicates a right to left cardiac shunt or a pulmonary arteriovenous fistula.

Haemorrhage
Cerebral hypoxaemia due to severe haemorrhage must be differentiated from respiratory failure, but usually a careful history and examination and haemoglobin estimation will establish the correct diagnosis.

Mental illness
Agitation, anxiety, restlessness and confusion may be signs of mental illness but before giving sedatives it is essential to be sure that they are not due to respiratory failure.

Coma
Carbon dioxide narcosis must be differentiated from coma due to other causes. Usually the history, physical examination and relevant investigations will establish the correct diagnosis (Table 16).

TREATMENT

The aims of treatment are to treat the cause of the respiratory failure, and at the same time maintain adequate oxygenation of the arterial blood, and if necessary reduce hypercapnia. Blood gas analysis is essential at the start of treatment and further analyses are required

Table 16 Differential diagnosis of coma.

	Common causes	Helpful investigations
C —	Carbon dioxide narcosis: ventilatory failure	Blood gas analysis
O —	Overdose: drugs	Serum levels
	alcohol	
M —	Metabolic disorders: diabetes mellitus	Blood glucose
	uraemia	Blood urea
	liver failure	Serum bilirubin
A —	'Apoplexy': cerebrovascular accident	Lumbar puncture
	head injury	Skull x-ray

to assess the effects of treatment. Treatment may be considered under the following headings:

Maintain a clear airway

It is absolutely imperative that the respiratory tract is kept free from excessive secretions. The methods used to remove secretions have been discussed in Chapter 6, and include assisted coughing, physiotherapy, bronchoscopy and aspiration via an endotracheal tube. If these methods fail tracheostomy may be necessary.

Oxygen

The principles of oxygen therapy and the methods of administration have been discussed in Chapter 6. It is essential when ordering oxygen to specify the method of administration, the concentration of oxygen, the flow rate and the humidification. In patients with acute respiratory failure the aim of oxygen therapy is to raise the P_aO_2 to at least 50 mmHg and preferably to 80 mmHg if this can be achieved without causing hypercapnia. If the P_aO_2 remains persistently below 40 mmHg despite intensive treatment, assisted ventilation may be necessary.

The concentration of oxygen is determined by the presence or absence of hypercapnia:

Hypoxaemia with a normal or low P_aCO_2 is treated with 40 to 60 per cent oxygen given by polymask or nasal catheter using a flow rate of 8l/min and adequate humidification.

Hypoxaemia with a raised P_aCO_2 is treated with 24 to 28 per cent oxygen by Ventimask. Treatment is begun with a 24 per cent mask, but this is substituted for a 28 per cent mask if the P_aO_2 remains below 50 mmHg, provided that the increased oxygen concentration does not aggravate the hypercapnia.

Avoidance of sedation

Drugs which may cause respiratory depression must be avoided. Opiates, barbiturates and tranquillizers should not be given to patients with respiratory failure unless the patient is being artificially ventilated.

Respiratory stimulants

The main value of respiratory stimulants is to rouse the drowsy hypercapnic patient temporarily so that he may be encouraged to cough. Intravenous nikethamide, 2 ml of a 25 per cent solution, will sometimes have this effect. Many physicians are confident that doxapram infusion, 0.5–4.0 mg per minute, is useful in stimulating respiration in hypercapnic respiratory failure.

Treatment of the cause of the respiratory failure

The treatment of the main causes of respiratory failure has been discussed in detail in the appropriate sections and may be summarized as follows:

Acute asthma: Corticosteroids, bronchodilators and antibiotics (p. 123).

Chronic bronchitis: Bronchodilators and antibiotics (p. 137).

Pneumonia: Antibiotics (p. 86).

Assisted ventilation

This is always indicated if a patient suddenly stops breathing, unless the patient is in the terminal stages of an incurable illness. In an emergency, mouth to mouth respiration or ventilation with an Ambu bag is lifesaving. As soon as possible the patient is intubated and connected to a ventilator. Cardiac arrest often accompanies respiratory arrest and requires appropriate treatment.

The other indications for assisted ventilation are difficult to define. In acute asthma assisted ventilation is *rarely* necessary but is indicated if the P_aO_2 is persistently below 40 mmHg. In asthma hypercapnia is a terminal sign, and if the P_aCO_2 remains above 50 mmHg after eight hours intensive treatment it may be necessary to ventilate the patient. Other signs which indicate the probable need for assisted ventilation include confusion, increasing heart rate, ineffective cough and exhaustion. Assisted ventilation is usually unnecessary in exacerbations of chronic bronchitis, but should be considered if the P_aO_2 remains below 40 mmHg and pH is less than 7.25 despite intensive treatment. The pH is a more accurate guide to the severity of acid-base disturbance than the P_aCO_2.

Other conditions in which ventilation may be necessary include barbiturate overdose, neuromuscular disorders and flail chest from multiple rib fractures. Artificial ventilation is rarely indicated in pneumonia.

Ventilation can be continued for some days through an endotracheal tube, but more prolonged ventilation is carried out through a tracheostomy. A patient who is being ventilated requires skilled medical and nursing attention and should be treated in an intensive care unit.

FURTHER READING

Bates D V Macklem, P T, Christie, R V 1971 Respiratory Function in Disease, 2nd edn. Philadelphia: Sauders.

Cotes J E 1979 Lung function, 3rd Edn. Blackwell Scientific Publications, Oxford

Crofton J, Douglas A 1981 Respiratory diseases. Blackwell Scientific Publications, Oxford

Flenley D C 1970 Respiratory failure. Scottish Medical Journal 15:61

Leading article 1981 Long term oxygen and advanced chronic bronchitis. Lancet i:701

Sykes M K, McNicol M W, Campbell E J M 1969 Respiratory failure. Blackwell Scientific Publications, Oxford

15

Pulmonary thromboembolism: pulmonary embolism and pulmonary infarction

DEFINITION

Pulmonary embolism occurs when an embolus, usually derived from a thrombus in the veins of the lower limb, lodges in the main pulmonary artery or its branches. *Pulmonary infarction* is the term used to describe the pathological changes which may develop in the lung after pulmonary embolism. Occasionally pulmonary infarction is the result of local thrombosis in the pulmonary artery. This group of related disorders is sometimes called pulmonary thromboembolism.

EPIDEMIOLOGY

The prevalence of thromboembolism in the community is unknown because frequently the embolic episode is minor and may not be diagnosed, or it may be confused with other diseases. Thromboembolism is the main cause of death in 5 per cent of all hospital patients. Routine autopsies have shown pulmonary emboli in 10 to 15 per cent of patients dying in hospital, while more detailed microscopic examinations have demonstrated recent or previous emboli in 50 per cent. For these reasons the doctor must be constantly aware of the possibility of pulmonary thromboembolism if the diagnosis is to be made with sufficient frequency.

With the exception of thromboembolism in pregnancy and in women taking oral contraceptives, the sex distribution is equal, and the disease is uncommon before the age of 40. Above this age the incidence increases with each decade.

AETIOLOGY

The majority of pulmonary emboli originate from thrombosis in the deep veins of the calf or the iliofemoral venous segment. Emboli may arise from the pelvic veins after pelvic surgery or parturition; occasionally embolism complicates thrombosis of superficial veins. About 10 per cent of pulmonary emboli originate from thrombosis in the right atrium secondary to atrial fibrillation, or from right ventricular mural thrombosis following myocardial infarction.

Emboli of non-thrombotic origin are uncommon. They include air, fat, malignant cells, amniotic fluid, trophoblast, parasites, vegetations and foreign material, e.g. cotton. Air embolism may occur during surgery on the head and neck or during injections into veins or hollow viscera. Fat embolism is common after trauma, especially after fractures of long bones, but rarely causes serious vascular obstruction. Amniotic fluid embolism is a rare and usually fatal complication of obstructed labour.

PATHOGENESIS AND PREDISPOSING CONDITIONS

Virchow suggested that the main factors responsible for venous thrombosis were damage to the vein wall, reduction in the rate of blood flow and increased coagulability of the blood. Once venous thrombosis has developed there is a risk of pulmonary embolism. Trauma to the vein, contraction of the leg muscles, straining or sudden change in the rate of blood flow may cause the thrombus to become detached from the vein wall. The thrombus may also fragment as a result of fibrinolysis.

Deep vein thrombosis
Venous thrombosis in the lower limbs is the commonest condition which predisposes to thrombo-embolism and it is important to review the clinical features of this condition. The main symptom is calf pain, and on examination the calf may be swollen and tender. Sometimes the thrombosed vein can be felt as a tender, thickened cord. Forcible dorsiflexion of the foot may produce calf pain (Homans' sign). Swelling of the calf may be detected only by careful measurement and comparison with the unaffected leg. The temperature of the affected leg may be higher or lower than that of the other leg. An important and frequently overlooked sign is unilateral ankle oedema. Sometimes this is the only sign of venous thrombosis, and unilateral ankle oedema of recent onset should always be regarded with suspicion.

The presence of these findings is variable and physical signs are absent in 50 per cent of patients with deep vein thrombosis. Investigations for detecting venous thrombosis include phlebography, the injection of ^{125}I labelled fibrinogen and the ultrasound technique.

Trauma
Trauma to the lower limbs, especially fracture of the hip, is associ-

ated with a high incidence of venous thrombosis and embolism. Trauma damages the vein wall and interferes with venous return.

Immobilization

Venous stasis due to immobilization is one of the principal factors responsible for deep vein thrombosis and pulmonary embolism. This is of particular importance in elderly, debilitated patients and in surgical and maternity cases. People who undertake long car or plane journeys and those who sit watching television for long periods are at increased risk of thromboembolism.

Obesity

A significant proportion of patients who develop thromboembolism are overweight but the reason for this association is not known.

Surgery

The precise incidence of postoperative thromboembolism is unknown but almost certainly it occurs more often than is suspected clinically. Usually embolism is secondary to venous thrombosis and special techniques have demonstrated deep vein thrombosis in 30 per cent of postoperative patients. Thrombosis is most common after abdominal surgery and in most instances it occurs during or immediately after the operation. Immobility, reduced fibrinolytic activity and increase in platelet numbers and adhesiveness are the main factors responsible for postoperative thromboembolism.

Pregnancy and the puerperium

The incidence of thromboembolism is increased in pregnancy and the puerperium and in some countries it is the commonest cause of maternal mortality. Thromboembolism usually follows deep vein thrombosis which is due to venous stasis, increase in clotting factors and decrease in fibrinolysins. Thromboembolism is commoner during the puerperium than during pregnancy and is more likely to occur in older multiparous women who have an operative delivery. It is also more frequent in patients in whom lactation is inhibited than in those who breast feed their babies. This may be due partly to oestrogens used to suppress lactation.

Oral contraceptives

The risk of thromboembolism was found to be increased sixfold in healthy women on oral contraceptives. It is the oestrogen rather than the progesterone component of these tablets which is responsible, and it affects clotting factors and platelet function. Lower oestrogen 'pills' have since been introduced.

Congestive heart failure
Peripheral venous stasis in cardiac failure may result in deep vein thrombosis and subsequent embolism. Pulmonary venous congestion predisposes to the development of pulmonary infarction after pulmonary embolism.

Myocardial infarction
Thromboembolism follows acute myocardial infarction in 5 per cent of patients.

Blood diseases
Polycythaemia vera predisposes to thromboembolism as a result of increased blood viscosity. Thromboembolism may follow splenectomy due to increase in platelet numbers and stickiness. It is of interest that thromboembolism is less common in people with blood group O than in those with other blood groups.

Malignancy
Thromboembolism is more common in patients with malignancy, particularly carcinoma of the pancreas, and may be due to release of thromboplastins into the circulation.

PATHOLOGY AND FUNCTIONAL ABNORMALITY

The size of the embolus determines its point of impaction in the pulmonary circulation and this influences the pathological findings and the severity of the haemodynamic disturbance.

The lung has a double blood supply through the pulmonary and bronchial arteries and pulmonary embolism does not cause infarction of the lung provided the bronchial circulation is adequate. After obstruction of the main pulmonary artery the bronchial arteries dilate and there is increased bronchial artery blood flow. Following obstruction of a branch of the pulmonary artery, interpulmonary arterial anastomoses develop between the branches of the affected artery and adjacent intact branches. These collateral channels also help to prevent infarction. Pulmonary congestion impedes the collateral circulation and contributes to the development of pulmonary infarction.

Emboli are often multiple, bilateral and recurrent and these factors also determine the structural and functional effects of thromboembolism. Multiple small emboli are more common than a single large embolus and 80 per cent of these emboli lodge in the lower lobes, the right more commonly than the left. This distribution is due to better perfusion of the lower lobes than the upper lobes. Selective streaming of blood to the right lower lobe in early systole accounts for the increased incidence of emboli and infarcts in this lobe although emboli are commonly bilateral.

Thromboembolism may be classified into three categories depending on the size of the embolus, the adequacy of the collateral circulation, and whether the emboli are mulitple or recurrent.

1. Massive pulmonary embolism

This occurs when a large embolus lodges in the right or left pulmonary arteries or straddles the bifurcation of the main pulmonary trunk (Fig. 23). Massive embolism causes a sudden fall in left ventricular filling resulting in decreased cardiac output and hypotension. The obstruction to blood flow causes acute right ventricular failure. Death may occur within minutes or hours if more than two thirds of the pulmonary blood flow is suddenly reduced.

Following massive embolism there is compensatory tachycardia, hyperventilation and tachypnoea. Embolism causes reduced perfusion of the lung and increase in the physiological dead space. Also there is reduced ventilation of regions of the lung adjacent to those deprived of blood flow, and this causes venous admixture resulting in hypoxaemia. Severe hypoxaemia causes metabolic acidosis. The P_aCO_2 falls as a result of hyperventilation. In patients who survive, the embolus undergoes lysis or becomes recanalized.

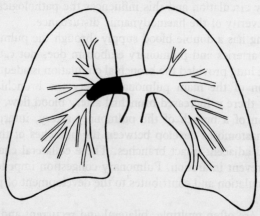

Fig. 23 Pathogenesis of massive pulmonary embolism: Obstruction of the right main pulmonary artery.

2. Pulmonary infarction

Infarction occurs if an embolus obstructs one of the larger branches

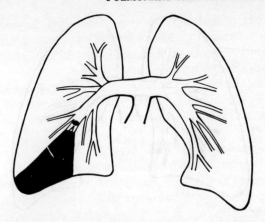

Fig. 24 Pathogenesis of pulmonary infarction: Obstruction of a medium-sized branch of the right pulmonary artery.

of the pulmonary artery and the collateral circulation is inadequate (Fig. 24). Ischaemic necrosis of the alveolar capillaries is followed by haemorrhage into the lung from the collateral circulation and by necrosis of the lung parenchyma. The physiological changes which accompany a large pulmonary infarct are similar to those which follow massive embolism, but the haemodynamic disturbance is less severe.

Eventually the infarct becomes organized and is replaced by a fibrous scar. An infarct frequently involves the pleural surface of the lung and is often accompanied by fibrinous pleurisy or small pleural effusion. Occasionally an infarct becomes infected, either because the embolus contains bacteria or because infection reaches the infarct through the bronchi or blood stream. In these cases a lung abscess may develop.

Lung scans and pulmonary angiography show that perfusion returns almost to normal in about 50 per cent of patients after embolism or infarction. Restoration of perfusion starts within a few days of the vascular occlusion and is usually maximal after four weeks, but may continue to improve during the next three months.

3. Recurrent obstructive pulmonary thromboembolism (obliterative pulmonary hypertension)

Small pulmonary emboli are unlikely to cause symptoms of embolism or infarction, but when they are numerous and recurrent they produce pulmonary hypertension if two thirds of the pulmonary vascular bed is obliterated (Fig. 25). The small arteries and arterioles are occluded by thrombus and by intimal proliferation,

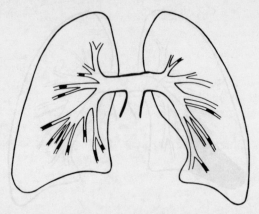

Fig. 25 Pathogenesis of recurrent obstructive pulmonary thromboembolism: Recurrent obstruction of multiple small branches of the pulmonary arteries.

and eventually compensatory right ventricular hypertrophy develops.

Pulmonary artery thrombosis may arise de novo in patients with impaired pulmonary blood flow due to cardiac failure, chronic lung disease or bronchial carcinoma, but in most cases pulmonary artery thrombosis results from thrombosis around an existing pulmonary embolus.

CLINICAL FEATURES AND INVESTIGATIONS

Massive pulmonary embolism

Clinical features

Massive pulmonary embolism occurs most commonly in surgical patients, usually during the second postoperative week, and in patients with chronic medical illnesses. Massive embolism is usually unexpected, although in retrospect it is not uncommon to find that the patient had transient fever, dyspnoea, tachycardia or chest pain due to a minor embolic episode which passed unrecognized.

The onset of massive pulmonary embolism is often dramatic and the patient may collapse and die within minutes. *Sudden severe central chest pain* and *breathlessness* are common.

Physical examination. The extreme respiratory distress is more sudden in onset and more severe than that seen in other emergencies, and is accompanied by signs of shock: pallor, rapid weak pulse, hypotension, cold extremities and sweating. Elevation of the jugular venous pressure, gallop rhythm and accentuation of the pulmonary second sound are common findings. Examination of the lungs usually shows no abnormality and evidence of deep vein thrombosis is detected in less 50 per cent of patients.

Investigations

Chest radiograph. This may show enlargement of the main pulmonary arteries or loss of vascular markings on the affected side, but these abnormalities are rarely obvious in a portable film.

Electrocardiograph. The ECG may show changes which are of diagnostic value and is also helpful in excluding cardiac disease. Tachycardia and low voltage waves are usually present. Abnormal patterns include T wave inversion in the right precordial leads, a dominant S wave in lead I accompanied by a Q wave and inverted T wave in lead III ($S_3 Q_3 T_3$ pattern) and right bundle branch block. These findings indicate right ventricular strain. A normal ECG does not exclude a diagnosis of pulmonary embolism.

Blood gas analysis. In suspected embolism, blood gas analysis is helpful. Hypoxaemia and hypocapnia, accompanied by severe metabolic acidosis, are compatible with a diagnosis of massive embolism.

Pulmonary scanning. The diagnosis of massive pulmonary embolism is confirmed by pulmonary scanning. Massive embolism causes gross reduction of pulmonary perfusion and this finding in association with a normal chest radiograph is diagnostic. Often the defects in perfusion are multiple and more extensive than would be suspected clinically or radiographically. If the lung scan is normal a diagnosis of massive embolism is most unlikely.

Pulmonary angiography. Angiography localizes the site of massive embolus but is not without risk and is usually indicated only when surgery is contemplated.

Pulmonary infarction

Clinical features

Pulmonary infarction may be preceded by symptoms suggestive of pulmonary embolism. The patient may complain of transient faintness or breathlessness, but these symptoms are not as severe as in massive embolism and are frequently overlooked by both patient and clinician. The classical triad of symptoms consists of *pleuritic pain, sudden dyspnoea* and *haemoptysis* but these features occur in less than 50 per cent of all patients with this condition. Pleuritic pain or haemoptysis is usually the first symptom, and when associated with deep vein thrombosis is sufficient evidence on which to make a clinical diagnosis of pulmonary infarction. Sudden dyspnoea accompanied by pleuritic pain should also suggest the possibility of pulmonary infarction, particularly when these symptoms arise under circumstances which predispose to thromboembolism. Recurrent attacks of pleuritic pain, breathlessness or haemoptysis occurring within some days of each other are also characteristic of infarction. Cough and sputum are not features of infarction but may be present if the patient has unrelated infection such as chronic bronchitis.

Physical examination. The commonest physical signs over a pulmonary infarct are dull percussion note, reduced breath sounds, coarse crepitations and pleural rub. The latter is the most helpful sign. Large infarcts may produce signs of consolidation. Frequently the patient has a low grade fever or tachycardia. Bilateral symptoms and signs are suggestive of pulmonary infarction.

Evidence of a source of embolism should always be sought in patients with possible infarction and the legs should be examined carefully. Signs of deep vein thrombosis are absent in 50 per cent of cases but this should not dissuade the physician from making a diagnosis of pulmonary infarction.

Investigations

Chest radiograph. The radiographic appearances of pulmonary infarction are non-specific. Commonly an infarct appears as an ill-defined opacity in the lower zone. Elevation of the hemidiaphragm frequently occurs on the affected side and a small pleural effusion may be present. A horizontal or curved linear opacity, several centimetres long, often appears in the periphery of the lower zone (Fig. 26). Bilateral radiographic changes in suspicious circumstances make the diagnosis virtually certain.

Peripheral blood. Polymorph leucocytosis and elevated ESR may occur in infarction but are also common in other diseases.

Pulmonary scanning. With the advent of radioisotope investigations it was hoped that pulmonary scanning would prove to be the ultimate technique for establishing a diagnosis of pulmonary infarction. Unfortunately this has not proved to be the case. Diminished pulmonary perfusion occurs in pulmonary infarction, but similar patterns are seen in pneumonia, bronchial carcinoma and other diseases which may be confused clinically and radiographically with infarction. Despite this disadvantage pulmonary scanning may assist diagnosis when it shows defects in perfusion in parts of the lung which appear normal on the plain radiograph. Provided the patient has no airways obstruction it is probable that the reduced perfusion is due to infarction. Concomitant ventilation scans aid the interpretation of the perfusion scan, especially in patients with airways obstruction.

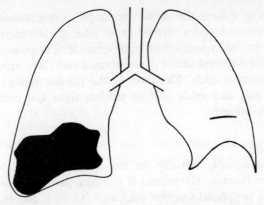

Fig. 26 Radiographic appearance of bilateral pulmonary infarction showing an ill-defined opacity on the right and a linear opacity and elevation of the diaphragm on the left.

Electrocardiograph. The ECG may show transient T wave inversion over the right precordial leads but does not provide information of diagnostic value.

Enzyme studies. Elevated serum bilirubin and lactic dehydrogenase levels sometimes develop in pulmonary infarction but are not a consistent finding, and since lactic dehydrogenase levels may rise in pneumonia, carcinoma and cardiac failure, enzyme studies are of limited diagnostic value.

Leg scanning. Since pulmonary infarction is usually secondary to deep vein thrombosis demonstration of deep vein thrombosis increases the likelihood that the patient's symptoms are due to infarction.

Recurrent obstructive pulmonary thromboembolism

Clinical features
The main symptoms of recurrent obstructive pulmonary thromboembolism are progressive dyspnoea and fatigue. The patient may also complain of attacks of syncope, chest pain and haemoptysis.

It is important to consider obliterative pulmonary hypertension in any patient with unexplained dyspnoea, chest pain or haemoptysis, particularly if there is a past history of puerperal or postoperative venous thrombosis. The onset and progression of the disease are insidious and the diagnosis is frequently overlooked until the patient has severe pulmonary hypertension.

Physical examination. The clinical signs of pulmonary hypertension are absent in the early stages but become obvious with progressive obliteration of the pulmonary vascular bed. There is a prominent 'a' wave in the jugular venous pulse, due to vigorous right atrial contraction and a systolic heave near the left sternal border produced by the hypertrophied right ventricle. The pulmonary component of the second sound is accentuated and there may be a pulmonary ejection click. Elevation of the jugular venous pressure, hepatomegaly and ankle oedema are late signs and indicate right ventricular failure.

Investigations

Chest radiograph. Initially the radiograph is normal but in the later stages there is enlargement of the main pulmonary arteries and loss of the peripheral vascular markings. There is also enlargement of the right ventricle and right atrium.

Electrocardiograph. When pulmonary hypertension is established, the ECG shows signs of right ventricular and right atrial hypertrophy and T wave inversion in the right precordial leads.

Blood gas analysis; pulmonary function tests. Blood gas analysis shows reduction of P_aCO_2. The hypoxaemia is worsened by exercise and improved by breathing high concentrations of oxygen. Exercise causes dyspnoea and hyperventilation disproportionate to the work load. Ventilation tests are normal, which is in striking contrast to the severity of the dyspnoea.

Cardiac catheterization. This may be necessary to confirm the diagnosis of pulmonary hypertension and to exclude disease of the left side of the heart such as mitral stenosis.

Pulmonary scanning; pulmonary angiography. These investigations are of limited value because they may fail to demonstrate obstruction of the smaller pulmonary arteries which are the vessels usually involved in this condition.

DIFFERENTIAL DIAGNOSIS
Massive pulmonary embolism

Spontaneous pneumothorax; pulmonary collapse
These conditions may mimic massive embolism but can be readily excluded by the physical and radiographic findings.

Myocardial infarction
This is the most common problem in differential diagnosis. The ECG usually shows evidence of myocardial infarction and the diagnosis is confirmed by finding elevated transaminase levels.

Acute haemorrhage
It is usually obvious when the circulatory collapse is due to acute blood loss, but the diagnosis may be difficult if the bleeding is due to a ruptured ectopic pregnancy.

Bacteraemic shock
Peritonitis, urinary unfection or septicaemia may cause circulatory collapse, but a careful history and examination should provide a clue to the correct aetiology. The most reliable differentiating sign is the jugular venous pressure, which is low in bacterial shock and increased in massive pulmonary embolism.

Pulmonary infarction

Pneumonia
It is often difficult to distinguish pulmonary infarction from pneumonia. Cough, sputum and fever favour pneumonia, and isolation of bacteria from the sputum is further evidence of an infective aetiology. In some cases it is impossible to distinguish pneumonia from infarction and it may be necessary to treat the patient with antibiotics and anticoagulants.

Bronchial carcinoma
This should be suspected if there is persistent haemoptysis or cough, or if finger clubbing is present. Sputum cytology and bronchoscopy may be necessary to exclude bronchial carcinoma.

Tuberculosis
The duration of symptoms is usually longer than in infarction and there may be a history of weight loss, night sweats and contact with tuberculosis. Tuberculosis mainly involves the upper lobes while infarction is more common in the lower lobes.

Pulmonary collapse
Postoperative pulmonary collapse causes sudden breathlessness and chest pain but can be diagnosed from the chest radiograph.

Recurrent obstructive pulmonary thromboembolism

Cardiac disease and chronic lung disease
Mitral stenosis, chronic bronchitis, emphysema and pulmonary fibrosis must be excluded as the cause of the pulmonary hypertension. A careful history and examination in conjunction with relevant investigations should facilitate this differentiation. Rarely, pulmo-

nary hypertension may be caused by tumour embolism, particularly choriocarcinoma.

Idiopathic pulmonary hypertension

This diagnosis has been given to certain patients with progressive pulmonary hypertension of unknown cause, but in retrospect it seems likely that most of these cases were due to thromboembolism. The diagnosis of idiopathic pulmonary hypertension should never be accepted without a prolonged trial of anticoagulant therapy in case thromboembolism is present.

TREATMENT

Massive pulmonary embolism

The treatment of massive pulmonary embolism includes the use of oxygen in high concentration, morphine, thrombolytic drugs, anticoagulants and in certain cases, surgery. The patient's progress should be carefully monitored.

Thrombolytic drugs such as streptokinase may cause lysis of pulmonary emboli, while anticoagulants prevent further thrombosis in the pulmonary arterial circulation. Anticoagulants also prevent further embolic episodes by reducing the likelihood of extension of the thrombotic process in the leg or pelvic veins. The best method of treatment is uncertain, although streptokinase is being used increasingly as initial treatment in preference to anticoagulants.

Streptokinase therapy

Before starting treatment hydrocortisone or an antihistamine is given to prevent hypersensitivity reactions. A loading dose of streptokinase, 600 000 units I. V., is given over 30 minutes and maintenance doses of 100 000 units are infused hourly for 72 hours. The dose is controlled by estimation of the thrombin clotting time. Heparin is then given for one week followed by warfarin for 3 to 6 months. Streptokinase therapy must not be repeated until antibody levels fall, usually a matter of 3 to 6 months.

Anticoagulant therapy

Heparin is the alternative method of treatment. Usually a loading dose of 10 000 units is given intravenously followed by constant infusion of 10 000 units 6 hourly for the first 24 hours. Further doses are determined by daily estimations of the whole blood coagulation time; the therapeutic range is 15 to 25 minutes. Heparin is continued for 1 to 2 weeks, followed by oral warfarin for a total of 3 to 6 months. Warfarin should be commenced two days before stopping heparin, with a loading dose of 30 mg on the first day and 10 mg on the second day; subsequent doses depend on the prothrombin time which is kept at 2 to 3 times the normal level.

Embolectomy
Early this century Trendelenburg showed that it was technically possible to remove massive pulmonary emboli, and since the development of cardiopulmonary bypass there have been numerous reports of successful pulmonary embolectomy. This operation still has a high mortality rate but may be lifesaving in patients with more than 75 per cent vascular occlusion, who are at risk of dying within 24 hours, or who show continued deterioration during thrombolytic or anticoagulant therapy. Before surgery it is essential to establish the diagnosis by angiography.

Pulmonary infarction

Anticoagulant therapy
Pulmonary infarction is treated with heparin for two days, using the same dose used in the treatment of pulmonary embolism. At the same time warfarin is started and is usually given for 6–12 weeks. If pneumonia cannot be differentiated from infarction, ampicillin should be given as well as anticoagulants.

Femoral vein ligation or vena caval ligation or plication has been advocated in patients in whom there is evidence of thrombosis in the leg or pelvic veins, and may be indicated if anticoagulants fail to prevent current embolism or if anticoagulants are contraindicated. Preoperative phlebography is essential to determine the exact site of thrombosis. Unfortunately these operations may be followed by thrombosis proximal to the ligation and are not widely practised.

Recurrent obstructive pulmonary thromboembolism

Recurrent pulmonary thromboembolism is treated with warfarin, which is continued indefinitely because of the risk of recurrent embolism and the development of intractible pulmonary hypertension.

PROGNOSIS

The mortality rate from massive pulmonary embolism is 50 per cent and death often occurs within hours of the embolic episode. Patients with pulmonary infarction usually recover provided anticoagulant therapy is started early. Recurrent obstructive pulmonary thromboembolism is frequently fatal because often the diagnosis is not made until there is severe pulmonary hypertension and right ventricular failure.

PREVENTION

Early mobilization after surgery and during the puerperium should be enforced and unnecessary immobilization during medical illnesses avoided. Prophylactic anticoagulant therapy with low-dose subcutaneous heparin or oral anticoagulants reduces the frequency of thromboembolism in predisposed patients. Elastic stockings are of doubtful value.

Early detection and treatment of deep vein thrombosis will reduce the incidence of thromboembolism. ^{125}I-fibrinogen, ultrasound or venography should be used when the diagnosis is in doubt, and anticoagulants should be given to all patients with deep vein thrombosis unless there is a definite contraindication.

FURTHER READING

Bell W R, Simon T L 1982 Current status of pulmonary thromboembolic disease: pathophysiology, diagnosis, prevention and treatment. American Heart Journal 103: 239

Browse N 1969 Deep vein thrombosis. British Medical Journal ii: 676

Goodwin J F, Harrison C V, Wilcken D E L 1963 Obliterative pulmonary hypertension and thrombo-embolism. British Medical Journal i: 701

Miller G A H 1976 Pulmonary thromboembolism. In: Lane, D I. (ed) Respiratory disease Tutorials in Postgraduate Medicine, Vol. 5, Heinemann, London

Miller G A H, Sutton G D, Kerr I H, Gibson R V, Honey M 1971 Comparison of streptokinase and heparin in treatment of isolated acute massive pulmonary embolism. British Medical Journal, i: 681

Pitney W R 1972 Clinical aspects of thromboembolism. Churchill Livingstone Edinburgh:

16

Bronchial carcinoma and other pulmonary tumours

BRONCHIAL CARCINOMA

Epidemiology

During the last 50 years there has been a worldwide increase in deaths from bronchial carcinoma. In Western countries bronchial carcinoma is the commonest neoplasm in males. Relatively few survive, and mortality rates give a good indication of the prevalence. In Britain the mortality rate in adult males is 100 per 100 000. Bronchial carcinoma occurs most commonly between the ages of 50 and 70, and men are affected four times more frequently than women.

Aetiology

Smoking
There seems little doubt that bronchial carcinoma is caused by cigarette smoking. More than 30 retrospective studies in 10 countries have demonstrated a direct relationship between the number of cigarettes smoked and the incidence of bronchial carcinoma. Prospective studies of nearly $1\frac{1}{2}$ million people have confirmed this finding. Among people who smoke 30 cigarettes per day the risk of dying from bronchial carcinoma is 30 times greaer than in non-smokers. Those who give up smoking permanently are much less likely to develop carcinoma after abstinence for 5 years. The risk of developing bronchial carcinoma is relatively low in pipe and cigar smokers. Experimental studies have now shown that mice and dogs made to inhale cigarette smoke develop lung cancer. The chief carcinogens in tobacco smoke are polycyclic aromatic hydrocarbons whose action is enhanced by phenols, fatty acid esters and free fatty acids. Nicotine is not a carcinogen.

Adenocarcinoma and alveolar cell carcinoma are not related to smoking, but these histological types are responsible for only a small proportion of all carcinomas.

Atmospheric pollution

Mortality from bronchial carcinoma is related to atmospheric pollution but its effect is small compared with the effect of cigarette smoking. Atmospheric pollution contributes to higher mortality rates in urban than rural dwellers. Polluted air contains hydrocarbons such as 3:4 benzpyrene which are carcinogenic.

Occupational factors

Bronchial carcinoma is more common in uranium miners, haematite miners, workers in the chromate industry, in nickel refining, in arsenic workers and in people with asbestosis. Cigarette smoking and asbestosis interact synergistically on the risk of developing bronchial carcinoma.

Pathology

Bronchial carcinoma may be classified into the following histological types:

Squamous cell carcinoma	45–50 per cent
Anaplastic carcinoma (small cell, oat cell)	35–40 per cent
Adenocarcinoma	15–20 per cent
Alveolar cell carcinoma	1–2 per cent

not relate to smoking.

Squamous cell carcinoma and anaplastic carcinoma arise from the surface of the bronchial epithelium. Anaplastic carcinoma has the worst prognosis due to its tendency to metastasize early. Adenocarcinoma develops from the mucous glands of the peripheral bronchi. Alveolar cell carcinoma arises from malignant change in type II alveolar cells. It is unifocal in origin but spreads by the air passages to give lesions in other parts of the lung.

About 50 per cent of tumours arise centrally from segmental or more proximal bronchi. The tumour is seldom more than a few centimetres in diameter on its mucosal surface but it causes bronchial irritation and ulceration which result in persistent cough and recurrent haemoptysis. Growth of the tumour into the lumen of the bronchus or infiltration of its wall produces partial bronchial obstruction which leads to retention of secretions and infection distal to the obstruction. This may result in pneumonia or lung abscess. A cavitated lesion may also result from ischaemic necrosis of the centre of the tumour. Complete bronchial obstruction causes pulmonary collapse. Symptoms also arise from local invasion of intrathoracic structures or from pressure on these structures by metastases in the mediastinal nodes. Lymphatic and haematogenous metastases are common. At autopsy 40 per cent of cases have metastases in the adrenal gland, liver, brain and bones. In only about 5 per cent of cases are metastases detected in each of these sites when the patient first presents. Radiography, organ scanning and other procedures are relatively unreliable in detecting small metastases.

The effects of bronchial carcinoma on respiratory function are relatively unimportant in comparison with its other effects. Impaired respiratory function is more often due to associated chronic bronchitis/emphysema than the tumour itself, although a large tumour or pulmonary collapse may cause reduced ventilation and perfusion in the affected region.

Clinical features

Bronchial carcinoma presents in a variety of ways and the onset of symptoms is often insidious. Usually the patient is first seen on account of specific respiratory symptoms or an acute respiratory infection. Sometimes the patient presents with general, non-specific symptoms but not infrequently he is asymptomatic and the lesion found incidentally on chest X-ray. Symptoms may also be due to local extension of the tumour, mediastinal metastases, or distant metastases. The figures quoted in the following section are mainly obtained from a review of 4000 patients with bronchial carcinoma managed in the Thoracic Surgical Unit in Edinburgh (Le Roux, 1968). The figures indicate the relative importance of the different manifestations of bronchial carcinoma.

Respiratory symptoms

Cough. This is a common symptom but often it is ignored by the patient or is attributed to smoking or to 'bronchitis'. When bronchial carcinoma develops in a patient with chronic bronchitis/emphysema the cough may become more frequent and the volume of sputum may increase. Persistent cough in an adult who is normally free of respiratory symptoms should always suggest the possibility of bronchial carcinoma.

Haemoptysis. In 60 per cent of patients there is a history of haemoptysis. Recurrent, slight blood streaking of the sputum is more common than a single profuse haemoptysis. Haemoptysis is frequently the first symptom, and in a smoker, haemoptysis should be regarded as presumptive evidence of bronchial carcinoma until proved otherwise.

Chest pain. Pain is less common than cough and haemoptysis. Bronchial carcinoma may cause three types of chest pain: pleuritic pain secondary to pneumonia or neoplastic involvement of the pleura, persistent deep aching chest pain caused by neoplastic invasion of the mediastinum, and localized chest wall pain and tenderness due to involvement of the ribs and intercostal nerves.

Dyspnoea. This is a variable symptom. Relatively sudden and severe breathlessness may occur if the tumour causes pulmonary collapse or if there is a large pleural effusion. Wheeze and stridor are uncommon unless the tumour involves the trachea or a bronchus close to the main carina. Breathlessness which becomes progressively more severe is a feature of lymphangitis carcinomatosa.

Acute respiratory infection

About 25 per cent of patients present with an acute respiratory infection. Symptoms include cough, purulent sputum, dyspnoea, haemoptysis and fever, and these may be due to acute bronchitis, pneumonia or lung abscess.

Pneumonia. This is commonly the first manifestation of bronchial carcinoma, and failure of pneumonia to clear after antibiotic treatment or recurrence of pneumonia in the same segment or lobe should always suggest the possibility of an underlying tumour.

Lung abscess. Bronchial carcinoma is a frequent cause of lung abscess.

General symptoms

About 10 per cent of patients present with general symptoms such as anorexia, weight loss, tiredness and ill health. Severe weight loss is a late symptom in bronchial carcinoma.

Asymptomatic, abnormal chest radiography

In 5 per cent of cases the patient is asymptomatic and the carcinoma is first detected as a result of a routine chest radiograph.

Features due to local extension of tumour or mediastinal metastases

Sometimes patients present with symptoms due to involvement of intrathoracic structures such as pleura, ribs, nerves, vessels or oesophagus by local extension of tumour or by mediastinal lymph node metastases.

Pleural effusion. In 10 per cent of patients pleural effusion develops as a result of neoplastic involvement of the pleura. Characteristically the effusion is bloodstained and reaccumulates rapidly after aspiration.

Rib involvement. This causes localized chest wall pain and tenderness.

Nerve involvement. Compression of the left recurrent laryngeal nerve causes hoarseness, while involvement of the phrenic nerve causes paralysis of the hemidiaphragm on the affected side which may produce breathlessness. These two manifestations occur in about 5 per cent of cases and are due to local extension of the tumour or to mediastinal lymph node metastases. Tumours in the apex of the lung occasionally involve the cervical sympathetic trunk, causing Horner's syndrome, or compress the brachial plexus giving pain, weakness and paraesthesiae in the arm and hand (Pancoast's tumour).

Superior vena caval obstruction. This occurs in 5 per cent of patients and is the result of compression of the superior vena cava by local extension of a tumour in the right upper lobe or by mediastinal metastases. The typical features include swelling and cyanosis of the face and neck, oedema of the arms, non pulsatile distension of the neck veins and dilated collateral veins over the upper chest.

Pericardial involvement. Involvement of the pericardium is uncommon but may give rise to cardiac arrhythmias or blood-stained pericardial effusion.

Oesophageal obstruction. Dysphagia due to oesophageal obstruction is an uncommon symptom.

Tracheal obstruction. This is also uncommon but may cause sudden stridor and severe dyspnoea.

Pulmonary lymphangitis carcinomatosa. Unilateral or bilateral lymphangitis carcinomatosa causes severe dyspnoea.

Features due to distant metastases

Cervical lymphadenopathy. In 15 per cent of patients the supraclavicular or retroclavicular lymph nodes are palpable. This is the commonest clinical sign of dissemination of bronchial carcinoma and usually occurs on the side of the lung lesion. Occasionally there is involvement of the contralateral nodes or of nodes on both sides of the neck. Axillary lymphadenopathy occurs only if the tumour invades the chest wall.

Cerebral metastases. About 3 per cent of patients present with cerebral metastases. Common symptoms include headache, fits, hemiplegia and personality changes.

Liver metastases. Hepatomegaly is rarely present when the patient is first examined.

Bone metastases. The ribs, vertebrae and pelvis are most frequently involved and pain is the commonest symptom.

Features due to non-metastatic syndromes

Occasionally patients present with features which cannot be attributed directly to local extension of tumour or to metastases. The mechanism responsible for these syndromes is uncertain; sometimes they precede radiographic evidence of the tumour.

Hypertrophic pulmonary osteoarthropathy. This occurs in 1 per cent of patients and is characterized by severe pain and swelling of the joints of the hands and feet, wrists and ankles, in association with finger clubbing. Radiographs show periosteal new bone formation at the distal end of the bones of the forearm and leg. An interesting feature is that the pain is relieved by resection of the neoplasm or by vagotomy.

Migratory thrombophlebitis. Migratory thrombosis of superficial veins is an occasional manifestation of bronchial carcinoma.

Neuromuscular syndromes. These syndromes include myopathy, myasthenia, peripheral neuropathy, encephalo-myelitis and sub-acute cerebellar degeneration.

Endocrine syndromes. Rarely the patient shows features which resemble Cushing's syndrome as a result of ectopic ACTH production by the tumour or its metastases. Inappropriate ADH secretion may produce symptomatic hyponatraemia, and ectopic parathormone secretion lead to hypercalcaemia. Hypoglycaemia and hyperglycaemia have been described in association with lung cancer.

Physical examination

Finger clubbing is a most important sign of bronchial carcinoma and is present in 60 per cent of patients.

Chest signs depend on the size of the tumour and its effect on intrathoracic structures. Many tumours produce no signs, but over a large tumour there may be dullness on percussion and reduced breath sounds. A fixed rhonchus is suggestive of tumour. Bronchial obstruction produces the signs of collapse while pleural involvement may give the signs of pleural effusion. Local extension of the tumour or metastases may cause localized rib tenderness, cervical lymph-adenopathy or signs of superior vena caval obstruction.

Investigations

Chest radiograph. Bronchial carcinoma may cause any of the following abnormalities.

A *dense hilar opacity* with an irregular margin is almost diagnostic of bronchial carcinoma. It may be due to the tumour itself but may also be caused by hilar lymph node metastases (Fig. 27).

A *solitary, circumscribed nodule* or 'coin' lesion of any size is commonly due to bronchial carcinoma (Fig. 28).

Localized ill defined shadowing in the lung field identical to that

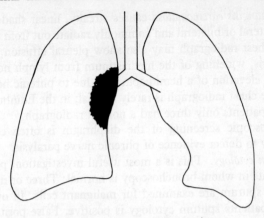

Fig. 27 Bronchial carcinoma producing a dense hilar opacity.

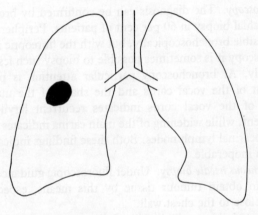

Fig. 28 Solitary circumscribed pulmonary nodule or 'coin' lesion. The differential diagnosis includes bronchial carcinoma, metastatic carcinoma, tuberculoma and benign tumours.

caused by lobular pneumonia is common. It may also represent pneumonia distal to a tumour (Fig. 10).

A *solitary cavitated lesion* similar in appearance to a simple lung abscess may be due to a cavitated bronchial carcinoma (Fig. 12). It may also represent a lung abscess secondary to pneumonia caused by infection of secretions distal to the bronchial obstruction. A neoplastic lung abscess often has thick irregular walls.

Collapse of a lobe or of the whole lung is common. Collapse produces a homgeneous opacity and signs of mediastinal displacement (Fig. 13–16).

Lymphangitis carcinomatosa causes streaky, linear shadows which are unilateral or bilateral and commonly radiate out from the hilum.

The chest radiograph may also show pleural effusion, osteolytic rib lesions, widening of the mediastinum from lymph node metastases, or elevation of a hemidiaphragm due to phrenic nerve paralysis. The chest radiograph is rarely normal; in the Edinburgh series of 4000 patients only three had a normal radiograph.

Fluoroscopic screening of the diaphragm is often carried out routinely to detect evidence of phrenic nerve paralysis.

Sputum cytology. This is a most useful investigation, particularly in patients in whom bronchoscopy is normal. Three or more specimens of sputum are examined for malignant cells. In over 80 per cent of patients sputum cytology is positive. False positives occur in less than 1 per cent of cases. Secretions obtained at bronchoscopy may also be examined for malignant cells.

Bronchoscopy. The diagnosis can be confirmed by bronchoscopy and bronchial biopsy in 60 per cent of patients. Peripheral tumours are not visible bronchoscopically, but with the fibreoptic instrument and fluorscopy it is sometimes possible to biopsy such lesions transbronchially. At bronchoscopy particular attention is paid to the movement of the vocal cords and the shape of the main carina. Paralysis of the vocal cords indicates recurrent laryngeal nerve involvement, while widening of the main carina indicates metastases in the subcarinal lymph nodes. Both these findings indicate that the tumour is inoperable.

Percutaneous needle biopsy. Under fluoroscopic guidance it is often possible to obtain tumour tissue by this means, especially from tumours close to the chest wall.

Scalene node biopsy. This will often establish the diagnosis if a palpable node is biopsied; blind biopsy is rarely positive.

Mediastinoscopy. Mediastinoscopy is sometimes carried out in patient with suspected bronchial carcinoma when sputum cytology and bronchosopy are normal. Mediastinoscopy is also carried out before thoracotomy for known carcinoma; demonstration of metastases in the mediastinal lymph nodes indicates that the tumour is inoperable.

Diagnostic thoracotomy. Sometimes the diagnosis cannot be confirmed by sputum cytology, bronchoscopy or lymph node biopsy and in such cases operation is often necessary. Indications for diagnostic thoracotomy include a persistent radiographic abnormality or pneumonia which has not resolved after several weeks' antibiotic treatment and physiotherapy. In these cases factors which favour early thoracotomy are a history of smoking, haemoptysis and finger clubbing.

Pleural aspiration and biopsy. Cytological examination of pleural fluid and pleural biopsy will establish the diagnosis in 60 per cent of malignant effusions.

Differential diagnosis
Bronchial carcinoma must be differentiated from other causes of cough, haemoptysis, finger clubbing or localized radiographic abnormality.

Pneumonia
This is an acute illness characterized by cough, purulent sputum and a radiographic abnormality which resolves with antibiotic treatment. Absence of definite radiographic improvement after treatment for 2 to 3 weeks should suggest the possibility of an underlying bronchial carcinoma, especially if the patient is a middle-aged smoker or has had haemoptysis. These are indications for bronchoscopy and cytological examination of the sputum.

Tuberculosis
A history of weight loss, night sweats and contact with tuberculosis accompanied by mottled shadowing in one or both upper lobes is more in keeping with a diagnosis of tuberculosis than bronchial carcinoma. In such circumstances the sputum must be examined for tubercle bacilli. Tuberculosis and bronchial carcinoma sometimes occur together.

Pulmonary infarction
This should be suspected if the illness is preceded by any of the conditions which predispose to thromboembolism or if there is evidence of deep vein thrombosis. The development of bilateral chest symptoms or signs also favours thromboembolism. Pulmonary scanning in bronchial carcinoma shows a perfusion defect at the site of the tumour which is similar to that seen in pulmonary infarction and is of little help in diagnosis. Usually the diagnosis of pulmonary infarction is made on clinical grounds (p. 157).

Chronic bronchitis/emphysema
These patients have an increased risk of developing bronchial carcinoma because the aetiology of both diseases is related to cigarette smoking. Increases in the severity of the cough, haemoptysis or the development of finger clubbing is an indication for an immediate chest radiograph.

Coin lesion

The differentiation of a peripheral circumscribed bronchial carcinoma from other 'coin' lesions is frequently difficult and resection is often necessary to establish the diagnosis (p. 178).

Treatment and prognosis

The prognosis of bronchial carcinoma is dismal and the overall 5 year survival rate is about 5 per cent. Patients with metastases die within a year of diagnosis. Squamous cell carcinoma has a better prognosis than anaplastic carcinoma. Surgery is generally the treatment of choice, but only 20 to 30 per cent of all patients are suitable for surgery. The 5-year survival rate after surgery is 25 to 30 per cent.

Surgery

Surgery involves lobectomy or pneumonectomy. Before thoracotomy it is imperative to exclude metastatic spread of the tumour. Careful clinical examination, including palpation of the supraclavicular lymph nodes, is essential. Palpable lymph nodes should be biopsied. Mediastinoscopy, barium swallow and screening of the diaphragm are used to detect evidence of mediastinal lymph node involvement. It is assumed that mediastinal metastases are present if the barium swallow shows oesophageal compression or if screening reveals paradoxical movement of the diaphragm. Pulmonary function is assessed by measurement of exercise tolerance, FEV_1 and blood gas analysis.

Contraindications to surgery

Advanced age. Over the age of 60 the operative mortality for lobectomy is 10 per cent and for pneumonectomy 20 per cent. Mortality is even higher in those over 70 and surgery is often inadvisable because the possible benefits are outweighed by the operative mortality and morbidity. The main causes of post-operative mortality are pneumonia, pulmonary embolism and myocardial infarction.

Inadequate pulmonary function. Surgery is contraindicated if the FEV_1 is less than 1.2 litres (lobectomy) or 1.8 litres (pneumonectomy). Elevation of the P_aCO_2 is a contraindication to surgery.

Local extension of tumour or metastases. Mediastinal or supraclavicular lymph node metastases, distant metastases, recurrent laryngeal or phrenic nerve paralysis, malignant pleural effusion and superior vena caval obstruction are contraindications to surgery.

Radiotherapy. Radical megavoltage radiotherapy is the alternative treatment when there is no evidence of metastases or chest wall involvement. Radical radiotherapy is contraindicated if metastases are present because it does not then prolong life. Palliative radiotherapy gives symptomatic relief in superior vena caval obstruction, tracheal obstruction, haemoptysis and bone pain.

Chemotherapy. Cytotoxic chemotherapy with a combination of drugs is probably better than radiotherapy for small cell carcinoma. Many regimens are currently being tested. In squamous cell carcinoma unsuitable for surgery cytotoxic chemotherapy can palliate symptoms but is more toxic and probably less effective than radiotherapy. Adenocarcinomas and alveolar cell carcinoma show little if any response to chemotherapy with presently available drugs. It is important to use adequate doses of chlorpromazine or metoclopramide to prevent or reduce nausea and vomiting. Alopecia should be anticipated by referral to a wig-fitter. Neutropenia, thrombocytopenia and anaemia are further complications and may limit therapy. Intrapleural injection of mustine 20 mg or tetracycline 500 mg sometimes prevents reaccumulation of malignant pleural effusions after pleural aspiration.

Laser therapy. Early reports suggest that lasers via the fibreoptic bronchoscope has a useful part to play in clearing radio-resistant, inoperable, intraluminal lesions obstructing a major bronchus or the trachea.

General management

It is extremely important to consider the patient as a whole. In elderly frail patients it is often more humane to advise no treatment rather than subject them to the discomforts of surgery, radiotherapy or chemotherapy.

Diazepam or chlorpromazine are given to relieve anxiety, and in patients with inoperable carcinoma prednisolone is given for its euphoric effect. Analgesics should be given in doses sufficient to relieve and prevent pain. Codeine and pholcodeine are useful in suppressing cough. Terminally, opiates must be used in adequate dosage and at appropriate time intervals. Comfort is then the main aim of management.

It is essential to appraise the patient's domestic and financial responsibilities and the doctor, the medical social worker and the church can provide emotional and material support for the patient and his family.

Prevention

Cigarette smoking is the major public health problem in Western countries and the continuing epidemic of bronchial carcinoma will decline only if cigarette consumption is drastically reduced. This may be achieved by fiscal means, antismoking campaigns, better health education, prohibition of cigarette advertisements and restrictions on smoking in public places. These measures depend largely upon government action. They will be successful if they convince the general public that smoking is an antisocial and lethal habit.

OTHER PULMONARY TUMOURS

Bronchial adenoma

This is the commonest benign neoplasm but its prevalance in relation to bronchial carcinoma is about 1:50. Although generally regarded as benign tumours they often show low grade malignancy and occasionally metastasize. Bronchial adenomas arise from the bronchial mucous glands and the commonest histological type is the carcinoid tumour.

Bronchial adenoma occurs most commonly around the age of 45 and women are affected as commonly as men. The majority of adenomas arise from the larger bronchi and cause cough, recurrent haemoptysis, unilateral wheezing, pneumonia and collapse.

Widespread metastases are rare but intrahepatic deposits may produce the carcinoid syndrome with attacks of flushing, tremor, fever, wheezing and diarrhoea. These attacks are probably related to release of 5-hydroxytryptamine (serotonin) and kinins.

The chest radiograph is often normal but may show pulmonary collapse. The diagnosis is made by bronchoscopy and biopsy. The majority of patients survive more than five years after resection.

Hamartoma

Hamartomas are composed of different tissues which normally occur in the lung but which are abnormally organized to form a tumour. Although they are developmental tumours they mainly occur after the age of 50. Unlike bronchial adenomas they usually arise in the periphery of the lung and are first detected as a 'coin' lesion in a routine chest radiograph. A hamartoma has a smooth outline, measures several centimetres in diameter and may show calcification. The diagnosis is made by resection which results in a cure.

Arteriovenous fistulae

These are uncommon vascular malformations which form a right to left shunt in the pulmonary capillary bed. The main features are central cyanosis, breathlessness, finger clubbing and polycythaemia. Sometimes a systolic murmur is heard over the fistula. The chest radiograph shows a rounded opacity a few centimetres in diameter in the periphery of the lung field. Vessels may be seen communicating with it. *Hereditary haemorrhagic telangiectasia* is present in 30 per cent of patients. The telangiectases involve the skin and mucous membranes and cause recurrent epistaxis and sometimes visceral bleeding. Pulmonary arteriovenous fistulae often cause haemoptysis, and for this reason surgical resection is sometimes recommended. Preoperative pulmonary angiography is essential to exclude multiple fistulae.

Pulmonary metastases

Metastases occur in the lungs in 30 per cent of all patients with malignancy. The most common sites of the primary tumour are the breast, stomach, colon, kidney, thyroid, bone and genital tract.

Pulmonary metastases do not usually cause respiratory symptoms, except lymphangitis carcinomatosa, which produces breathlessness which is insidious in onset and becomes progressively more severe. Sometimes there is history of previous malignancy or there are symptoms referable to the primary tumour.

Pulmonary metastases cause the following radiographic abnormalities: solitary nodule or 'coin' lesion, multiple nodules and lymphangitis carcinomatosa.

Coin lesions

Diagnosis is often difficult in patients with a solitary pulmonary nodule and the causes of 'coin' lesions are shown in Table 17. The radiographic features of the nodule may assist in diagnosis. Tomograms may show that the nodule has a clearly defined margin which is more in favour of a benign than a malignant lesion. Calcification within the nodule is more common in benign lesions, especially tuberculomas. Cavitation suggests the possibility of tuberculosis or a

Table 17   Causes of a solitary pulmonary nodule or 'coin' lesion

Common
  Bronchial carcinoma
  Metastatic carcinoma
  Tuberculoma

Uncommon
  Hamartoma
  Arteriovenous fistula
  Rheumatoid nodule
  Lung abscess
  Hydatid cyst

An apparent 'coin' lesion may be due to a skin lesion or an artefact cavitated bronchial carcinoma. Despite these differences it is often impossible to determine the aetiology of the lesion, and investigations such as bronchoscopy and bacteriological and cytological examination of the sputum are of little diagnostic value. In the majority of patients with a solitary nodule it is necessary to carry out surgical resection to establish the diagnosis and to exclude carcinoma.

Before thoracotomy for a solitary nodule it is essential to examine the chest wall for a skin lesion such as a papilloma. It is also important to examine previous chest radiographs. If it can be shown that the lesion has been present for more than two years and is unchanged in size it can be assumed to be benign. In these circumstances thoracotomy is not indicated but serial radiographs should be taken every six months.

FURTHER READING

Azzopardi J C, Freeman E, Poole G 1970 Endocrine and metabolic disorders in bronchial carcinoma. British Medical Journal iv:528

Bignall J R 1966 Early diagnosis of bronchial carcinoma. British Medical Journal i:341

Durrant K R, Ellis F, Black J M, Berry R J, Ridehalgh F R Hamilton W S 1971 Comparison of treatment policies in inoperable bronchial carcinoma. Lancet i:715

Fox W, Scadding J G 1973 Medical research council comparative trial of surgery and radiotherapy for primary treatment of small-celled or oat-celled carcinoma of bronchus, ten year tollow-up. Lancet iii:63

Fraser R G, Paré J A P 1979 Diagnosis of diseases of the chest. 2nd ed Saunders, Philadelphia

Geddes D M 1979 The natural history of lung cancer: a review based on rates of tumour growth. British Journal of Diseases of the Chest 73:1

Lawson R M, Ramanthanan L, Hurley G, Hinson K W, Lennox S C 1976 Bronchial adenoma: review of an 18-year experience at the Brompton Hospital. Thorax 31:245

Le Roux B T 1959 Pulmonary arteriovenous fistulae. Quarterly Journal of Medicine 28:1

Le Roux, B T 1964 Pulmonary hamartomata. Thorax 19:236

Le Roux B T 1968 Bronchial carcinoma. Livingstone, Edinburgh

Levison V 1980 What is the best treatment for early operable small cell carcinoma of the bronchus? Thorax 35:721

Oswald N C, Hinson K F W, Canti G, Miller A B 1971 The diagnosis of primary lung cancer with special reference to sputum cytology. Thorax 26:623

Royal College of Physicians 1977 Smoking or health. Pitman, London

17

Mediastinal tumours

CLASSIFICATION

A large variety of tumours occur in the mediastinum. Some arise as developmental tumours of intrathoracic structures but the majority are due to involvement of the mediastinal lymph nodes by metastatic carcinoma or lymphoma. In addition, intrathoracic lesions such as an aortic aneurysm or intrathoracic thyroid may present as mediastinal tumours (Table 18).

CLINICAL FEATURES

The clinical features of mediastinal tumours depend upon the site and nature of the tumour and the mediastinal structures which it compresses or invades. Benign tumours often grow to a large size without causing symptoms and may be detected first by routine radiography. They usually have a clearly defined outline. Malignant tumours are likely to cause symptoms early because of invasion of vital structures. Often no abnormal signs are detected on examination of the chest.

Table 18   Classification of mediastinal tumours

Lymph node tumours
Metastatic carcinoma: bronchus, breast, bowel
Lymphoma e.g. Hodgkin's disease
Leukaemia

Developmental tumours and cysts
Neural tumour e.g. neurofibroma
Dermoid cyst
Teratoma
Thymoma
Pleuropericardial cyst
Bronchial cyst

Lesions acting as mediastinal tumours
Intrathoracic thyroid
Aortic aneurysm
Hiatus hernia

The clinical features may be summarized in relation to the structures which are involved:

Trachea: Cough, dyspnoea, stridor.

Bronchi: Cough, dyspnoea.

Oesophagus: Dysphagia.

Superior vena cava: Swelling and cyanosis of the face, neck and arms, non-pulsatile distension of the neck veins and distension of the superficial veins of the arms. Dilated anastamotic veins develop over the anterior chest wall and blood flows in a downward direction to reach the inferior vena cava.

Pericardium: Pericarditis, pericardial effusion.

Sympathetic trunk: Horner's dyndrome —ptosis, myosis, anhidrosis and enophthalmos on the affected side.

Phrenic nerve: hiccups, paralysis of the diaphragm.

Left recurrent laryngeal nerve: hoarseness, paralysis of the left vocal cord.

Features of different mediastinal tumours

Lymph node tumours

These are most commonly caused by metastases from bronchial carcinoma but may be due to metastases from neoplasm elsewhere or to lymphoma or leukaemia. Enlarged lymph nodes in the superior and anterior mediastinum may cause pressure symptoms. Weight loss is a prominent symptom in metastatic disease and fever is common in Hodgkin's disease. The chest radiograph shows a mediastinal mass and there may also be paratracheal node enlargement (Fig. 29).

Neural tumours

Neural tumours such as neurofibroma are one of the commonest mediastinal tumours. They arise from the sympathetic ganglia or intercostal nerves and lie in the paravertebral gutter. They may cause spinal cord compression and intercostal pain and may be associated with neurofibromatosis (von Recklinghausen's disease). In the lateral chest radiograph a neural tumour appears as a rounded dense opacity overlying the spine. Neural tumours sometimes undergo malignant change.

Dermoid cysts and teratomas

Dermoid cysts are composed mainly of tissues of ectodermal origin while teratomas contain tissues derived from all three germinal layers. These tumours may contain skin, hair, sebaceous glands, teeth, bone, cartilage, muscle and different types of epithelial tissue. Der-

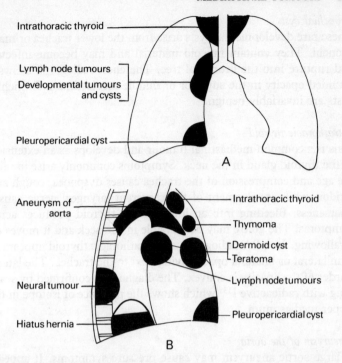

Fig. 29 Common sites of mediastinal tumours. (A) AP view; (B) Lateral view.

moid cysts and teratomas are usually symptomless. The chest radiograph shows a rounded homogeneous opacity in the anterior mediastinum; calcium and teeth may be seen within the opacity. These tumours may undergo malignant change.

Thymomas
Tumours of the thymus gland lie in the superior and anterior mediastinum and cause symptoms by pressure on the trachea, bronchi or superior vena cava, although frequently they are first detected by routine radiography. Thymomas may be associated with myasthenia gravis and hypogammaglobulinaemia. Thymomas are locally invasive but rarely metastasize.

Pleuropericardial cysts
These cysts contain clear fluid and arise as developmental abnormalities of the pericardium. They do not cause symptoms and are benign. The radiograph shows an opacity with a smooth convex outer border in the right cardiophrenic angle.

Bronchial cysts

These rare developmental cysts arise from the lower trachea or main bronchi. They contain mucoid material and may become infected and rupture into the bronchial tree. The chest radiograph shows a rounded opacity in the superior or middle mediastinum. Bronchial cysts are invariably benign.

Intrathoracic thyroid

This is a common mediastinal tumour and develops as an extension of the thyroid gland in the neck. Symptoms commonly arise in middle age and compression of the trachea causes dyspnoea, cough and stridor, while involvement of the recurrent laryngeal nerve causes hoarseness. Bleeding into an intrathoracic thyroid produces acute symptoms. The goitre may be palpable in the neck and it moves on swallowing. In a PA radiograph an intrathoracic thyroid appears as a unilateral or bilateral opacity lying next to the trachea. The lateral border of the opacity is convex. The diagnosis is confirmed by scanning with radioactive I^{131} which shows the presence of isotope in the upper mediastinum.

Aneurysm of the aorta

A large aortic aneurysm may cause pressure symptoms. It appears as a smooth rounded swelling in the superior or middle mediastinum and may be seen to pulsate on screening. The wall of the aneurysm often contains calcium.

Hiatus hernia

The commonest type of hiatus hernia is caused by herniation of the stomach through the oesophageal foramen in the diaphragm. The PA radiograph shows a fluid level apparently lying within the heart, but the lateral radiograph shows that the fluid level is actually behind the heart. A barium meal confirms the diagnosis. Rarely a hiatus hernia arises through the ventral foramen of Morgagni, the foramen of Bochdalek, or a traumatic defect in the diaphragm.

INVESTIGATIONS

Determination of the exact site of a mediastinal tumour is of diagnostic help and may be established by lateral radiographs, tomography and screening. Computerised axial tomography, bronchoscopy, sputum cytology and mediastinoscopy are useful in the diagnosis of lymph node tumours.

Previous chest radiographs should be examined and if these show that the tumour has been present for many years and is unchanged in size, it is probably benign. Often thoracotomy is necessary to establish the diagnosis and to exclude malignancy.

TREATMENT

There is usually no effective treatment for lymph node tumours due to metastic carcinoma, but secondaries from oat cell carcinoma or breast carcinoma sometimes regress with radiotherapy and/or chemotherapy. Lymphoma and leukaemia often respond to radiotherapy and/or chemotherapy. Neural tumours, dermoid cysts, teratomas and thymomas are resected because of the risk of malignant degeneration. An intrathoracic thyroid is resected because of the danger of tracheal compression.

FURTHER READING

Hinshaw H C, Murray A F 1980 Diseases of the chest, 4th Edn. Saunders, Philadelphia

Le Roux B T, Dodds T C 1968 A second portfolio of chest radiographs. E & S Livingstone, Edinburgh

18

Pulmonary tuberculosis

EPIDEMIOLOGY

Man has been afflicted with tuberculosis since the beginning of civilization and evidence of the disease has even been detected in Egyptian mummies entombed hundreds of years before the birth of Christ. Tuberculosis remains the most important infectious disease in the world.

In Europe the prevalence of tuberculosis started to decline during the 19th century due to improved living standards. During the past three decades antituberculosis drugs and BCG have had a dramatic effect on morbidity and mortality in affluent countries. In Britain the notification rate of new cases is 16 per 100 000 and the mortality rate is 3 per 100 000. Although these rates are comparatively low, tuberculosis is not a rare disease, and the total number of deaths attributed to tuberculosis greatly exceeds those due to all other infectious diseases. In 20 per cent of fatal cases the diagnosis is first made after death and the physician must constantly think of tuberculosis in order to ensure prompt diagnosis and treatment.

In Western countries tuberculosis occurs most commonly in middle-aged and elderly men. The highest rates in Britain occur in immigrants from India, Pakistan and Bangladesh. Native races such as North American Indians and Canadian Eskimos show high rates. In the developing countries of Africa and Asia tuberculosis is an enormous problem. Many millions have active tuberculosis and it is the major single cause of death.

Predisposing factors
The following immunological and environmental factors predispose to the development of tuberculosis but it is often difficult to determine the relative importance of each because several factors may coexist.

Racial origin. Races which have relatively recently come into contact with tuberculosis for the first time show increased susceptibility.

This partly explains the high prevalance of tuberculosis in North American Indians and Eskimos.

Living conditions. Overcrowded housing conditions facilitate the spread of tuberculosis and it is more common in the lower socio-economic groups and close-knit Asian immigrant households.

Nutrition. Malnutrition may be partly responsible for the increased prevalence of tuberculosis in developing countries.

Diseases. *Alcoholism, diabetes mellitus* and *silicosis* increase individual susceptibility to tuberculosis. Tuberculosis is also more common in patients with *immunological disorders* such as leukaemia and Hodgkin's disease. *Gastrectomy* predisposes to tuberculosis.

Smoking. Tuberculosis is more common in heavy smokers than in non-smokers.

Corticosteroids. Long term treatment with corticosteroids and other immuno-suppressive drugs lowers resistance to tuberculosis, facilitates the spread of the disease and can cause reactivation of quiescent lesions.

AETIOLOGY

In 1882 Koch discovered the bacillus responsible for tuberculosis. It belongs to the genus *Mycobacterium* and the following species cause disease in man:

M. tuberculosis. This is the cause of virtually all cases of human tuberculosis. The disease is spread by droplets of sputum, and infected cases act as the source of infection. Patients showing acid fast bacilli in sputum smears are highly infectious, but when the sputum is positive only on culture the risk of transmission is relatively slight.

M. bovis. This bacillus causes bovine tuberculosis and is now rarely responsible for human disease because tuberculosis has been almost eradicated from cattle in Western countries and milk is pasteurized. Tuberculosis cervical lymphadenitis and mesenteric lymphadenitis are occasionally seen in older people infected many years previously with *M. bovis*.

Atypical mycobacteria. These bacteria are usually saprophytes but occasionally they cause disease in man (p. 202).

BACTERIOLOGY AND IMMUNOLOGY

The diagnosis of tuberculosis is established bacteriologically when *M. tuberculosis* is isolated from sputum, urine, cerebrospinal fluid pleural fluid or biopsy tissue. Usually three specimens of sputum are collected on successive days. Specimens may be sent by post to the laboratory. Laryngeal swabs or gastric washings are examined if sputum is not available.

Sputum smears stained by the Ziehl-Neelsen method are examined microscopically for acid fast bacilli which appear as tiny, refractile red rods.

Sputum culture is a more sensitive method for detection of tubercle bacilli and is necessary for identification of acid fast bacilli seen in smears. *M. tuberculosis* is a slow growing organism and the culture requires 4 to 10 weeks incubation. Demonstration of tubercle bacilli in smear or on culture indicates the presence of active tuberculosis.

Sensitivity tests are carried out if tubercle bacilli are isolated and take 4 to 6 weeks. One commonly used method estimates the minimum concentration of antituberculosis drug required to inhibit growth of the patient's organism compared with a standard test organism. The result is expressed as a resistance ratio.

Tuberculin tests

About 4 to 6 weeks after infection with *M. tuberculosis* the patient becomes hypersensitive to tuberculoprotein, a component of the tubercle bacillus, and an intradermal injection of tuberculoprotein causes induration at the injection site. This is a delayed hypersensitivity reaction mediated by lymphocytes (Type IV reaction) and is the basis of the tuberculin test.

The Mantoux test and the Heaf test are the two most widely used tuberculin tests. A purified protein derivative of tuberculoprotein (PPD) is used more commonly than Koch's Old Tuberculin.

Mantoux test. An intradermal injection of 0.1 ml PPD or Old Tuberculin is given on the flexor aspect of the forearm. For epidermiological purposes the concentration used is 5 tuberculin units (5TU) but in diagnosis and in the examination of contacts 10TU are used. If negative the test may be repeated with 100TU. The diameter of induration at the injection site is measured after 48 to 72 hours. Induration 10 mm or more in diameter indicates a positive reaction. Erythema at the site of the injection is not significant.

Heaf test. This is a multiple puncture test which is easy to perform and it is often used for epidemiological surveys. It is read after 3 to 6 days. Induration for four or more of the six puncture sites indicates a positive reaction. The reaction is graded from I to IV according to the amount of induration.

Tine test. This is a multiple puncture test in which tuberculin is incorporated on the prongs of a disposable unit. The tine test is equivalent to a 5TU Mantoux test.

Interpretation of the tuberculin test. The size of the reaction must be correlated with the concentration of tuberculin employed; a positive reaction to 10TU is more significant than a positive reaction to 100TU. A positive tuberculin test is evidence of previous or present infection with mycobacteria, but does not necessarily signify infection with *M. tuberculosis* nor does it indicate active disease. Small reactions may be caused by anonymous mycobacteria or previous BCG vaccination; reactions over 10 mm induration with the Mantoux test or Heaf grades II to IV are usually due to *M. tuberculosis*. Large reactions are common in active tuberculosis but activity can only be proven by bacteriological studies.

Tuberculosis is unlikely to be present if the tuberculin test is negative, although negative reactions sometimes occur in severely ill patients and in miliary tuberculosis. Corticosteroids suppress the tuberculin reaction and it is often negative in sarcoidosis and lymphoma.

Non-specific reactions. The significance of low grade tuberculin senstitivity is difficult to intepret. Weakly positive Mantoux and Heaf tests may be cross reactions due to infection with anonymous mycobacteria which are antigenically similar to *M. tuberculosis*. When this is the case, skin tests with antigens prepared from anonymous mycobacteria will usually produce strongly positive reactions.

Epidemiological studies. The tuberculin test is used to assess the prevalence of tuberculosis in the community. In Britain 10 per cent of 13-year-old children are tuberculin positive compared with 75 per cent of children in India. Decline in the proportion of tuberculin positive persons indicates a falling prevalence of tuberculosis.

Mass vaccination campaigns with BCG are often carried out without preliminary tuberculin testing. Where tuberculin tests are carried out, tuberculin negative children are given BCG while tuberculin positive children are assumed to have been naturally infected and are not vaccinated. Contacts of patients with tuberculosis are routinely tuberculin tested to determine those who are tuberculin negative and should be given BCG, and those who are tuberculin positive and require further assessment to exclude active tuberculosis. Use of the tuberculin test for case finding is only of value in a community where tuberculosis prevalence is low.

PATHOLOGY AND PATHOGENESIS

The tubercle is the characteristic lesion of tuberculosis and gives the disease its name. It consists of a concentric collection of epithelioid cells surrounded by lymphocytes and fibroblasts, and may contain

Langhans' giant cells and acid fast bacilli. The centre of the tubercle often becomes necrotic. This process is called *caseation* and distinguishes the tubercle of tuberculosis from the follicle of sarcoidosis. In adults the caseous material may be discharged into a bronchus leaving a cavity in the parenchyma of the lung. Tuberculous lesions heal by fibrosis and often become calcified. *Cavitation* and *calcification* are characteristic features of tuberculosis.

Primary tuberculosis

Primary tuberculosis is the name given to the initial tuberculous infection. It usually occurs in childhood and in the majority of cases the lung is the site of the primary infection. The initial lesion is an area of pneumonia in the periphery of the mid or lower zones of the lung parenchyma. This is followed by tubercle formation. The infection spreads to the hilar lymph nodes which enlarge as a result of tubercle formation and caseation. These two components, the peripheral parenchymal lesion and the proximal lymph node lesion, form the primary tuberculous complex. Similar changes occur if the primary infection is caused by the bovine bacillus although the portal of entry of infection is the tonsil or the small bowel, and the lymph nodes which are involved are the cervical or mesenteric.

When primary tuberculosis develops in adolescents or adults there is minimal lymph node involvement and the parenchymal lesion occurs in the upper lobes.

Fate of the primary complex

In the majority of cases the primary complex heals. Occasionally it is followed by pulmonary complications or haematogenous spread which may cause disease in other organs. Tubercle bacilli in the primary complex may lie dormant, and reactivation of infection at any time in the future results in postprimary pulmonary tuberculosis. Treatment of primary tuberculosis with antituberculosis drugs prevents these complications.

Pulmonary complications
These are most likely to occur within a year of the primary infection.
 Progressive pulmonary tuberculosis
Occasionally the primary complex doesn't heal and gives rise to postprimary pulmonary disease.
 Lobar collapse. This is due to bronchial obstruction caused by enlarged hilar lymph nodes or caseous material which has ruptured from lymph nodes into the bronchial lumen.
 Tuberculous pleurisy. Infection may spread via the lymphatics to

the pleura causing tuberculous pleural effusion (p. 253). The effusion is produced by a hypersensitivity reaction to tuberculoprotein due to the presence of tubercle bacilli in the pleural space.

Haematogenous spread

Tubercle bacilli in the primary complex may enter the bloodstream and become widely disseminated. This usually occurs within a year of the primary infection, although symptoms due to haematogenous spread may not appear until many years later.

Miliary tuberculosis. The main sites of miliary tuberculosis are the lungs, spleen, liver, lymph nodes, kidneys and meninges. Usually more than one site is involved and the disease may be acute or chronic.

Tuberculous meningitis. This develops as a result of rupture of a subcortical caseous focus into the subarachnoid space. It is not always accompanied by evidence of miliary tuberculosis elsewhere.

Bone and joint tuberculosis. This usually occurs within three years of primary infection and the joints most commonly affected are the spine, hip, knee or wrist.

Genito-urinary tuberculosis. Genito-urinary lesions appear five or more years after the primary infection. The infection begins in the kidney and spreads downwards to involve the ureter and bladder, and in the male the epididymis. Tuberculosis of the fallopian tubes is usually secondary to disease of the ovary or endometrium and may result in sterility.

Other sites involved by haematogenous spread include the pericardium, presenting as pericardial effusion or constrictive pericarditis, and the adrenal glands, resulting in Addison's disease.

Postprimary pulmonary tuberculosis

This is the commonest complication of primary tuberculosis and accounts for most cases of tuberculosis in adults. Usually it is the result of reactivation of infection which has occured in childhood or adolescence, but occasionally it is due to reinfection with tubercle bacilli. Adult tuberculosis differs from primary tuberculosis in the following ways: the lesion is usually situated in the upper lobes or sometimes the apical segment of the lower lobes; it is frequently bilateral, and cavitation is common.

PRIMARY PULMONARY TUBERCULOSIS

Clinical features

The majority of children do not develop symptoms and the infection passes unrecognized although occasionally the child suffers a mild febrile illness with cough, anorexia and malaise.

Physical examination. Usually there are no abnormal findings but signs of pulmonary collapse may be present if the primary complex causes bronchial obstruction. *Erythema nodosum* occasionally accompanies the primary infection and may be the only clinical evidence of primary tuberculosis. Erythema nodosum appears as bluish red, indurated, tender swellings on both legs (p. 207).

Investigations

Chest radiograph. In children the typical appearance of primary tuberculosis is unilateral hilar enlargement and a localized opacity in the periphery of the lung (Fig. 30), The two shadows may merge so that the lymph node and parenchymal components cannot be differentiated. These abnormalities resolve after some months, and within a year of the primary infection the radiograph may show spotty calcification in the draining lymph nodes and a speck of calcification at the site of the parenchymal lesion.

In adolescents and young adults there is usually no visible hilar lymphadenopathy and the only abnormality is mottled shadowing in the upper lobe which cannot be distinguished from postprimary tuberculosis. Sometimes the chest radiograph is normal in primary tuberculosis.

Tuberculin test. The tuberculin test becomes strongly positive about 6 weeks after the onset of the primary infection. If the tuberculin test is negative it is most unlikely that tuberculosis is present.

Bacteriological examination. The child seldom produces sputum and if tuberculosis is suspected it may be necessary to carry out gastric lavage.

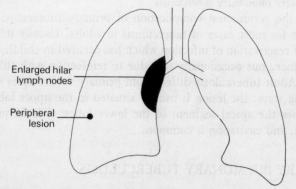

Enlarged hilar
lymph nodes

Peripheral
lesion

Fig. 30 Primary tuberculosis showing peripheral parenchymal lesion and proximal hilar lymph node enlargement.

Differential diagnosis

Primary tuberculosis must be differentiated from acute *upper respiratory tract infections* and *pneumonia*, and from disease such as *sarcoidosis* and *lymphoma* which cause hilar lymphadenopathy and erythema nodosum.

MILIARY TUBERCULOSIS

Clinical features

The clinical pattern of miliary tuberculosis has changed in countries where tuberculosis prevalence is low, and it is now more common in adults, especially those over the age of 50, than in children.

In *children and young adults* miliary tuberculosis is usually an *acute illness* with anorexia, malaise, weight loss, respiratory symptoms, fever, sweats, abnormal pain and sometimes meningitis. Meningitis causes headache, vomiting, neck stiffness and neurological signs. Choroidal tubercles are occasionally present and appear as yellowish, circular lesions in the optic fundus.

In *middle-aged and elderly adults* miliary tuberculosis is usually a more *chronic illness*. The onset is insidious and often the patient has been ill for several months before presentation. Because symptoms are frequently non-specific there may be delay in diagnosis. The main features of this cryptic form of miliary tuberculosis are *general ill-health*, anorexia, weight loss and fever. Other features include sweats, genito-urinary symptoms and signs, and sometimes meningitis. Respiratory symptoms are rare. Miliary tuberculosis should always be considered when these features occur in a patient with a past history or contact history of tuberculosis. Miliary tuberculosis may follow prolonged treatment with corticosteroids or immunosuppressive drugs and may complicate immunological disorders such as leukaemia.

Investigations

Chest radiograph. Miliary mottling is present in only 60 per cent of patients. In these cases the radiograph shows opacities 2 mm or less in diameter distributed diffusely throughout the lungs (Fig. 31). Occasionally there is pleural effusion. There may be evidence of previous primary or post primary tuberculosis, e.g. calcification of the hilar lymph nodes and focal calcification in the lung parenchyma or upper zone fibrosis and calcification. The chest radiograph is normal in 15 per cent of patients, the so-called cryptic miliary group.

Bacteriological examination. Every attempt should be made to obtain a bacteriological diagnosis by examination of sputum, gastric

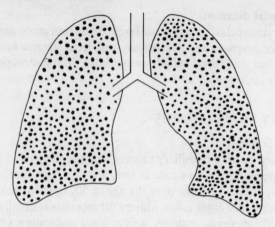

Fig. 31 Miliary tuberculosis. The differential diagnosis includes bronchopneumonia, sarcoidosis, pneumoconiosis, fibrosing alveolitis and lymphangitis carcinomatosa.

washings, urine or bone marrow. Sometimes it is not possible to confirm the diagnosis by bacteriological means. If the patient has symptoms of meningitis the cerebrospinal fluid is examined immediately. Cerebrospinal fluid which contains lymphocytes and has a low glucose concentration should be regarded as being due to tuberculous meningitis until proved otherwise.

Tuberculin test. The tuberculin test is sometimes initially negative, which may be misleading, although it usually becomes positive during the course of the illness.

Liver biopsy. If other investigations fail to substantiate the diagnosis, liver biopsy should be done, for it may reveal caseating granulomas or be positive on culture.

Lymph node biopsy. This may provide a histological or bacteriological diagnosis, especially in patients with lymphadenopathy.

Therapeutic trial. A therapeutic trial with isoniazid and ethambutol is a valuable diagnostic test in patients with persistent unexplained fever. Fever due to tuberculosis will usually subside within two weeks of starting treatment. Streptomycin or rifampicin are not given initially because they influence fever due to brucellosis and other bacterial infections.

Differential diagnosis
Miliary tuberculosis must be differentiated from other diseases which cause ill health, weight loss and fever, e.g. *malignancy, leukemia, lymphoma* and *chronic pyelonephritis*. Relevant investigations will usually provide the correct diagnosis, but differentiation from

leukaemia may be difficult, especially when it is complicated by miliary tuberculosis. Differentiation from other diseases which cause miliary mottling is not difficult; *sarcoidosis* and *pneumoconiosis* rarely cause weight loss and fever, while *bronchopneumonia* and *allergic alveolitis* cause acute respiratory symptoms. If bronchopneumonia cannot be excluded on clinical grounds ampicillin should be given while carrying out investigations.

POST-PRIMARY PULMONARY TUBERCULOSIS

Clinical features

Constant awareness of the possibility of tuberculosis is the key to correct diagnosis. The onset of the illness is usually gradual and often symptoms have been present for several months or longer before the patient seeks medical attention.

Persistent cough, haemoptysis, weight loss, night sweats and *malaise* are the classical symptoms of pulmonary tuberculosis. Any one of these symptoms should suggest the possibility of tuberculosis and the diagnosis is even more likely when they occur in combination. In this context a family history or contact history of tuberculosis, and the presence of environmental or immunological factors which predispose to tuberculosis, are highly significant.

The patient may present with apparent *pneumonia*; tuberculosis should always be considered if symptoms have been present for several weeks or if the radiographic abnormalities fail to resolve after antibiotic treatment.

Sometimes the patient is asymptomatic and the disease is first detected by a routine chest radiograph.

Physical examination. There may be evidence of weight loss and in patients with extensive tuberculosis finger clubbing and fever are common. Examination of the chest is frequently normal.

Investigations

Chest radiograph. A normal chest radiograph virtually excludes the presence of pulmonary tuberculosis. The typical radiographic abnormalities include patchy mottled shadows, cavitation and calcification predominantly involving the upper zones. A minimal lesion appears as soft apical shadowing (Fig. 32), while more severe disease causes extensive bilateral lesions with cavitation (Fig. 33). Tuberculosis is the commonest cause of a pulmonary cavity. Tomography may be used to confirm cavitation. In chronic tuberculosis there may be fibrosis with displacement of the trachea and mediastinum to the

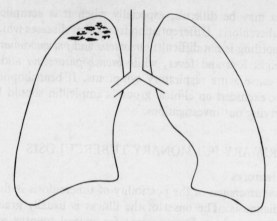

Fig. 32 Pulmonary tuberculosis. Minimal lesion causing apical shadowing.

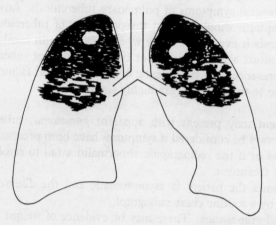

Fig. 33 Pulmonary tuberculosis. Extensive bilateral lesions with cavitation.

affected side. Occasionally a tuberculous cavity becomes blocked with caseous material giving rise to a circumscribed homogeneous opacity, 1 to 2 cm in diameter, which is called a tuberculoma (p. 178). Tomography may show calcification and satellite lesions.

Bacteriological examination. At least three specimens of sputum should be examined by smear and culture, and if sputum is unavailable laryngeal swabs or gastric contents should be examined.

Tuberculin test. The tuberculin test is usually strongly positive; active tuberculosis is unlikely if the tuberculin test is negative. However tuberculin hypersensitivity may be depressed in debilitated patients with extensive disease and in patients receiving cortico-steroids.

Peripheral blood. Anaemia may be present; often the white cell count and ESR are normal.

Differential diagnosis

Tuberculosis must be considered in any patient who presents with cough, haemoptysis, weight loss or night sweats, and in any patient with an abnormal chest radiograph, especially if this shows upper zone lesions, cavitation or calcification. The most common problems in differential diagnosis are pneumonia, pulmonary infarction and bronchial carcinoma.

Pneumonia. Usually the history is of short duration but some-times differentiation from tuberculosis is difficult. It is advisable to examine the sputum for tubercle bacilli in all patients with pneu-monia. Failure of pneumonia to respond to antibiotics should alert the physician to the possibility of tuberculosis.

Pulmonary infarction. This should be suspected when the condi-tions which predispose to pulmonary thromboembolism are present. Pulmonary infarction is an acute illness and does not cause weight loss or night sweats, and the radiographic abnormalities do not usually involve the upper zones.

Bronchial carcinoma. A localized dense opacity is more in favour of tumour than tuberculosis, especially if there is evidence of hilar enlargement. Sputum cytology and bronchoscopy may be necessary, especially if a thick walled irregular cavity is present. Occasionally bronchial carcinoma and tuberculosis co-exist, and thoracotomy may be necessary if the diagnosis is in doubt.

Chronic bronchitis. Persistent cough should never be attributed to chronic bronchitis or cigarette smoking unless tuberculosis has been excluded by chest radiography.

TREATMENT

Principles of chemotherapy

Crofton and his colleagues in Endinburgh first showed, by con-trolled clinical and bacteriological studies, that antituberculosis chemotherapy produces sputum conversion in 100 per cent of patients with active pulmonary tuberculosis. The patient can be assured of cure provided the following criteria are fulfilled:

1. The infecting organism is sensitive to the drugs which are given.

2. The drugs are given in the correct dose, correct combination and for adequate time.

3. The patient takes the drugs with the utmost regularity.

The dramatic success of Crofton's régime was due to the fact that patients were given triple chemotherapy with streptomycin, isoniazid and PAS (para-aminosalicylic acid).

Treatment with a single antituberculosis drug usually results in the development of resistant organisms. Although single drug therapy initially eliminates the sensitive bacilli, naturally-occurring resistant mutants rapidly multiply until the whole bacterial population is resistant. If two drugs are given, each suppresses the mutants which are naturally resistant to the other drug as well as eliminating the bacilli which are sensitive to both drugs.

Primary drug resistance

This is a term used when a patient, who has never received antituberculosis chemotherapy, is primarily infected with tubercle bacilli which are resistant to one or more drugs. The prevalence of primary resistance to one drug is about 1 per cent in Britain, North America and Australia. In some of the developing countries, where chemotherapy has been inadequately controlled, the incidence of primary drug resistance is as high as 10 per cent.

Secondary (acquired) drug resistance

This term is used when resistant tubercle bacilli are isolated from a patient who was initially infected with sensitive bacilli but whose organisms have subsequently become resistant as a result of inadequate chemotherapy. Secondary drug resistance results from the use of inadequate drug regimens which allow the emergence of resistant mutants. Patients with secondary drug resistance form the infector pool from which the majority of patients with primary resistance are infected.

A treatment regimen which employs three drugs will prevent the emergence of naturally resistant mutants and will also be effective if the patient's bacilli are primarily resistant to one of the drugs.

Before starting treatment

It is vitally important to enquire whether the patient has been treated previously, and if so, to obtain details of this treatment and of previous bacteriological studies. If the patient has been treated it should be assumed that the organism might be resistant to one or more of the drugs given. Likewise it is important to obtain similar information about the source case, and if the patient has been in contact with a person with known drug resistance it should be assumed that the patient may have resistant organisms. In both instances the patient should be treated as a case of possible drug resistant tuberculosis until the results of current sensitivity tests become available (p. 199), although it is usually possible to predict with reasonable certainty the sensitivity pattern of the organism.

For the reasons given above it is essential that treatment with antituberculosis drugs is supervised by specially trained physicians and nurses.

Chemotherapy

Triple therapy is always given initially and the combination of rifampicin, isoniazid and ethambutol is widely used (Table 19).

Triple therapy with rifampicin, isoniazid and ethambutol is given for 2 months and then rifampicin and isoniazid are continued until the patient has had a total of 9 months treatment. Regimens not containing both rifampicin and isoniazid should be continued for a total of 18 months. Continuation chemotherapy regimens should always contain at least two effective antituberculosis drugs.

Initial treatment is often given in hospital in order to prevent spread of the disease by smear positive patients, to ensure that the patient is taking and tolerating the drugs, and to educate the patient in the principles of treatment. The patient may be treated at home if the disease is minimal and the direct smear is negative, and the social conditions are good. Enforced bed rest is unnecessary.

Culture conversion to negative occurs within 3 months in 80–90

Table 19 Drugs used in the treatment of tuberculosis

Drug	Method of administration	Daily dose	Side effects
Rifampicin*	Capsule	450–600 mg	Liver toxicity enzyme induction
Isoniazid	Tablet	200–300 mg	Peripheral neuropathy
Ethambutol	Tablet	25 mg/kg (for first 2 months) 15 mg/kg (after 2 months)	Retrobulbar neuropathy
Streptomycin	I.M.	0.75 to 1.0 g	Vertigo
Pyrazinamide	Tablet	1.5 to 2.5 g	Hyperuricaemia, rashes
Thiacetazone	Tablet	150 mg	Nausea, vomiting, liver toxicity, blood dyscrasias

* Commonly given in a combined preparation with isoniazid.
† Available in a combined preparation with isoniazid.

per cent of patients and in 5 to 6 months in the remainder. Infectivity wanes rapidly after the start of chemotherapy and after 2 to 3 weeks even smear-positive patients may be regarded as noninfectious. For the first 3 weeks of treatment patients who were positive on direct smear should avoid young children and immunosuppressed patients but isolation and barrier nursing are unnecessary.

Out-patient supervision of chemotherapy is essential and the patient attends a clinic every two months or so in order to check clinical, bacteriological and radiographic progress. At each clinic attendance the patient's urine can be tested for rifampicin or isoniazid. It is helpful for the district nurse to call at the patient's home to check that treatment is being taken regularly.

If the patient is considered unreliable fully supervised regimens such as the Madras regimen are used for domiciliary treatment. This consists of twice weekly streptomycin, 1 g, with isoniazid, both of which are given by the district nurse. A high dose of isoniazid (15 mg/kg) is used; in addition pyridoxine, 10 mg, is given to prevent isoniazid toxicity. If the patient fails to attend for treatment the doctor is notified.

Regimens of four drugs for 2 months with continuation of rifampicin and isoniazid to a total of 6 months are under clinical trial, as are various intermittent oral regimens.

If streptomycin is given to patients over the age of 40 years the dose is reduced to 0.75 g daily. In patients with impaired renal function the dose is adjusted according to the results of serum streptomycin levels. Streptomycin should be stopped immediately if the patient develops vertigo; it is then necessary to give a lower dose of streptomycin or to use an alternative drug.

Ethambutol may cause retrobulbar neuropathy and patients must be told to report any reduction in visual acuity or red/green discrimination and to stop the drug immediately. Rifampicin colours the sputum, tears and urine reddish-brown but this is of no consequence. Thrombocytopenia may occur with high dose intermittent rifampicin. Pyrazinamide in doses of 2.5 g/day or less is an effective and safe drug. Isoniazid rarely causes side effects.

Hypersensitivity reactions

Hypersensitivity reactions to modern triple chemotherapy are rare, in contrast to the 10 per cent of patients who used to experience such reactions to PAS and streptomycin in the 2nd to 5th weeks of treatment. The manifestations of hypersensitivity are fever and rash, and the drugs most commonly responsible are rifampicin and streptomycin. Reactions to isoniazid are rare, and when they occur they are usually accompanied by hypersensitivity to the other two drugs.

Treatment is stopped as soon as a hypersensitivity reaction develops; after the reaction has subsided a test dose of each drug is given in turn to determine which is responsible. The drug responsible for the reaction will produce fever or rash. If the patient is hypersensitive to one drug, treatment is continued with the other two drugs and another drug added until the drug sensitivities of the organisms are available. If it is imperative that the patient be desensitised this can be achieved by starting with a small dose and thereafter increasing the dose daily over a period of 1 to 2 weeks. Desensitization is usually accomplished without difficulty but occasionally it is necessary to give corticosteroids at the same time. During desensitization it is essential that the patient is not given one drug alone since resistance may develop within two weeks.

Drug resistant tuberculosis
Patients who are known or suspected to have been infected with organisms resistant to one or more of the standard drugs are given at least three drugs to which the organisms is known to be or can be assumed to be sensitive (p. 197). Sensitivity tests are used for the selection of effective drugs. Ethambutol and rifampicin are commonly used for drug resistant cases and it may be necessary to include reserve drugs such as ethionamide, prothionamide, cycloserine, capreomycin or kanamycin. The incidence of side effects from reserve drugs is relatively high.

Corticosteroids
Corticosteroids and potassium supplements are used in patients who are moribund with extensive tuberculosis. Prednisolone, 60 mg daily, is usually used in the treatment of tuberculous meningitis adhesions. Corticosteroids are sometimes used during drug desensitization and as replacement therapy in patients with Addison's disease. Corticosteroids will hasten the resolution of tuberculous pleural effusion. Corticosteroids should never be given to a patient with tuberculosis without adequate cover with antituberculosis drugs.

Surgery
It is doubtful if there is any indication for surgery in the treatment of pulmonary tuberculosis, but occasionally resection is carried out in patients with resistant organisms. Surgery is no substitute for

chemotherapy and it is essential that effective drug treatment is continued after resection.

PREVENTION

The methods used for prevention of tuberculosis in different countries depend on its prevalence and the economic resources of the country. In many countries the tuberculosis services work in consultation with expert bodies such as the Medical Research Council and WHO.

Treatment of active cases

The best means of prevention is to reduce the size of the infector pool by adequate treatment of known patients with active tuberculosis. In economically developing countries domiciliary chemotherapy is widely used to minimize the cost of large-scale therapeutic programmes, and trials are in progress to discover drug regimens which are effective, inexpensive and readily tolerated.

Case finding

The unknown pool of infection must be detected and treated. Tuberculin testing, radiography and sputum examination are used for case finding among contacts of recently diagnosed patients with active tuberculosis and for regular case finding surveys in the community.

Contacts. In Britain, close contacts of recently diagnosed patients are tuberculin tested and have a chest radiograph. Those who are tuberculin negative are given BCG and discharged, as are those known to have had BCG previously, unless the chest radiograph is abnormal. If the index case was positive on direct smear tuberculin positive close contacts who have not previously had BCG should have repeat chest radiographs at one and two years. If the radiograph is abnormal sputum should be examined for tubercle bacilli by smear and culture. If the index case was negative on direct smear it is not necessary to repeat the contact examinations at one and two years except perhaps in the Asian immigrant groups. Screening of casual contacts is not usually worthwhile.

Community surveys. Miniature radiography has helped to reduce the prevalence of tuberculosis in developed countries. The yield of infected cases detected by regular mass radiography is now relatively small, and surveys are mainly confined to people who are particularly susceptible to infection, and to occupational groups which are likely to infect others, eg: persons living in poor institutions and prisons, alcoholics, public transport workers, school teachers, nurses, dentists and doctors.

Direct smear examination of sputum is the cheapest and most effective method of community case finding in developing countries with a high prevalence of tuberculosis.

Tuberculin testing is of limited value for case finding in countries where tuberculosis is prevalent or where BCG is widely used.

BCG vaccination (Bacille-Calmette-Guérin)

BCG vaccination has contributed considerably to the decline in tuberculosis and provides an 80 per cent protection rate in young adults if a satisfactory vaccine is employed. The policy regarding BCG vaccination varies from country to country according to the epidemiological situation. Where there is a high prevalence, mass vaccination is appropriate, whereas in areas of low prevalence BCG vaccination may be applicable only to persons at risk such as nurses, doctors and laboratory technicians. Large-scale community vaccination is carried out in Europe and in developing countries. In Britain 13-year-old children are tuberculin tested and those found to be tuberculin negative are given BCG but this practice is likely to become unrewarding by the late 1980s.

Chemoprophylaxis

In some European countries and in North America chemoprophylaxis with isoniazid, 300 mg daily, is given to people considered to be at risk of developing active tuberculosis. These include: persons with radiographic abnormalities due to inactive tuberculosis who have not previously been given chemotherapy, recent tuberculin converters with normal chest radiographs, children with strongly positive tuberculin tests and individuals with inactive tuberculosis receiving long term treatment with corticosteroids or immunosuppressive drugs.

In Britain chemoprophylaxis has not been widely used because of the risk that it may lead to the development of isoniazid resistant bacilli. However this risk is slight, and because chemoprophylaxis reduces the chance of reactivation of tuberculosis it is now being given more frequently.

MYCETOMA

Occasionally tuberculous cavities fail to close after adequate chemotherapy, and about 20 per cent of patients with a residual cavity develop a mycetoma. A mycetoma is so named because it is a fungus ball composed of mycelia. It usually arises as a result of saprophytic colonization of the cavity with *A. fumigatus*, in which case it is sometimes called an aspergilloma. Occasionally other fungi are responsible for a mycetoma.

Patients with a mycetoma often have a chronic cough and suffer recurrent haemoptysis which may be severe. The chest radiograph shows a dense irregularly rounded opacity surrounded with a halo of radiotranslucency (Fig. 34). There is usually fibrosis elsewhere in the lung as a result of previous tuberculosis. Precipitins to *A. fumigatus* are commonly present and this test is used to confirm the diagnosis. Aspergillus may be isolated from the sputum. Treatment is not usually necessary although occasionally a mycetoma is resected on account of severe haemoptysis.

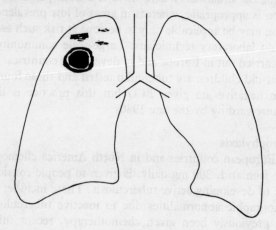

Fig. 34 Mycetoma. A halo of translucency surrounds a fungus ball in a post-tuberculous cavity.

ATYPICAL MYCOBACTERIA

Atypical (anonymous) mycobacteria are common saprophytes in the environment, and although they are responsible for a relatively high prevalence of low-grade tuberculin hypersensitivity they seldom cause clinical disease. In Britain atypical mycobacteria are isolated from 1.5 per cent of patients whose radiographs show apparent pulmonary tuberculosis. Atypical mycobacteria most frequently cause disease in the Southern States of the U.S.A. and in Australia.

Atypical mycobacteria are classified by their bacteriological characteristics which differ from those of *M. tuberculosis*. The main pathogenic atypical mycobacteria are *M. kansasii*, *M. avium-intracellulare* and *M. xenopi*. They cause disease which is clinically and radiographically indistinguishable from pulmonary tuberculosis. Pulmonary disease occurs more commonly in patients with current industrial dust exposure. Atypical mycobacteria are often resistant in vitro to antituberculosis drugs but good results are nevertheless obtained with 15 months of rifampicin and ethambutol (M. kansasii) and 2 years of rifampicin, isoniazid and ethambutol (M. avium-intracellulare).

FURTHER READING

British Medical Journal 1980 Isolation of patients with pulmonary tuberculosis. Leading article i:980

British Medical Journal 1980 BCG in Britain. Leading article 281:825

British Thoracic and Tuberculosis Association 1975 Short course chemotherapy in pulmonary tuberculosis. Lancet i:119

British Thoracic Association 1980 Short course chemotherapy in pulmonary tuberculosis: Lancet i:1182

British Thoracic Association 1982 A controlled trial of six months chemotherapy in pulmonary tuberculosis. American Review of Respiratory Diseases, 126:460

Crofton J, Douglas A 1981 Respiratory Diseases 3rd edn. Blackwell Oxford

Fox W 1981 Whither short course chemotherapy? British Journal of Diseases of the Chest 75:331

Ross J D, Horne N W 1983 Modern drug treatment of tuberculosis 6th edn. Chest and Heart Association, London

19

Sarcoidosis

DEFINITION

Sarcoidosis is a systemic granulomatous disease of unknown aetiology which may affect the hilar lymph nodes, lungs, skin, superficial lymph nodes, eyes, liver, spleen, nervous system, bones and heart.

EPIDEMIOLOGY

Sarcoidosis is of world-wide distribution. In Europe, North America and Australia the prevalence of pulmonary sarcoidosis is about 20 per 100 000. The highest incidence is in the 20 to 40 age group, and women are affected slightly more often than men.

AETIOLOGY

In many respects sarcoidosis resembles tuberculosis but *M. tuberculosis* cannot be isolated from the lesions; the tuberculin test is often negative, BCG does not afford protection and antituberculosis drugs are ineffective. There is no proof that sarcoidosis is due to infection with atypical mycobacteria, fungi or viruses, and theories that sarcoidosis is a reaction to pine pollen and hair sprays have not been confirmed.

Patients with sarcoidosis show altered immunological reactivity. Delayed hypersensitivity reactions are depressed as shown by depression of tuberculin hypersensitivity and negative skin tests to common antigens such as mumps and *C. albicans*. This is due to impaired activity of cellular antibodies. Circulating antibody production is normal and the serum globulins may be increased.

It seems probable that individuals with altered immunological reactivity develop sarcoidosis in response to certain agents. It may be a reaction to a specific transmissible agent because innoculation of human sarcoid tissue into mice results in a sarcoid reaction at the site of injection.

PATHOLOGY AND FUNCTIONAL ABNORMALITY

Non caseating epithelioid cell follicles are the common histological feature of sarcoidosis and are a constant finding whatever the site of the disease. These follicles or granulomas are composed of focal collections of epithelioid cells, small numbers of lymphocytes and a few giant cells of Langhans' type. Unlike the tubercles of tuberculosis, sarcoid follicles do not undergo caseation; their reticulin architecture is retained and initially they are all at the same stage of development. Inclusion bodies occur in the giant cells but this finding is not peculiar to sarcoidosis. Sarcoid granulomas usually resolve spontaneously but if they persist they are replaced by hyaline fibrosis. Fibrosis is a feature of chronic sarcoidosis.

The histological features of sarcoid granulomas are not specific and granulomas wth a similar appearance occur in histoplasmosis, brucellosis, leprosy and berylliosis as well as tuberculosis. Local sarcoid tissue reactions occasionally develop in lymph nodes draining a carcinoma or as a local lymph node response to zirconium which is present in deodorant sticks. These reactions are unlikely to be confused with sarcoidosis since the clinical manifestations of the disease are absent.

In the thorax, sarcoid granulomas occur in the alveolar walls, bronchi, lymphatics and lymph nodes. Sarcoidosis of the parenchyma of the lung may be followed by widespread interstitial fibrosis. Granulomas are often present in the skin, superficial lymph nodes, eyes, liver and spleen. The nervous system, kidneys, heart and bones are less frequently involved. Pleural effusion is rare.

The functional effects of sarcoidosis depend upon the site and the extent of the lesions and the degree of fibrosis. In the eyes and nervous system relatively localized lesions impair function. In the lung the commonest and earliest abnormality is reduction in diffusing capacity. Extensive pulmonary fibrosis causes reduction in total lung capacity, a restrictive ventilatory abnormality and decreased pulmonary compliance. Hypoxaemia may occur, although in mild cases this is present only after exercise.

CLINICAL FEATURES

The patient may present with symptoms and signs due to sarcoidosis in one more sites and the course of the disease may be subacute or chronic (Table 20).

Table 20 Clinical features of subacute and chronic sarcoidosis

	Subacute	Chronic
Duration	<2 years	>2 years
Age	<30 years	>30 years
Onset	Sudden	Insidious
Lungs	Hilar lymphadenopathy	Pulmonary opacities
	Pulmonary opacities	Pulmonary fibrosis
Skin	Erythema nodosum	Plaques
	Maculopapular eruptions	Lupus pernio
Lymphadenopathy	Present	Absent
Eyes	Acute uveitis	Chronic uveitis
	Conjunctivitis	Glaucoma, blindness
Bone cysts	Absent	Present
Kveim test	Positive	May be negative
Spontaneous remission	Common	Uncommon
Prognosis	Good	Poor

Bilateral hilar lymphadenopathy

This present in 80 per cent of patients and is frequently the first sign of sarcoidosis. Bilateral hilar lymphadenopathy is often accompanied by erythema nodosum, arthralgia and uveitis. Sometimes the paratracheal nodes are also enlarged. Occasionally unilateral hilar enlargement is detected before the development of bilateral lymphadenopathy. Hilar lymphadenopathy may be accompanied by parenchymal lesions but usually these are minimal. Bilateral hilar lymphadenopathy rarely causes respiratory symptoms and is often detected by routine chest radiography in apparently healthy young adults. In the majority of cases it resolves spontaneously.

Pulmonary sarcoidosis

Pulmonary opacities occur in 40 per cent of patients. They accompany the hilar lymphadenopathy or may develop independently. Initially there are no symptoms but if fibrosis occurs the patient develops breathlessness and cough. Progressive fibrosis causes increasing dyspnoea and disability. Pulmonary sarcoidosis does not cause finger clubbing and examination of the chest is usually normal.

Thoracic sarcoidosis is conventionally classified as Stage I if there is just hilar adenopathy; Stage II: hilar adenopathy + pulmonary opacities; Stage III: pulmonary opacities only.

Skin

The skin is affected in 20 per cent of patients and the commonest lesion is erythema nodosum. This is an early manifestation of sarcoidosis. Rounded, red, tender nodules appear on both shins. The nodules are 1 to 6 cm in diameter and persist for several weeks; as they fade they resemble bruises. Erythema nodosum is invariably accompanied by bilateral hilar lymphadenopathy and often by malaise, arthralgia and fever.

Other skin lesions include pink coloured nodules and plaques and sometimes these develop in old scars. Lupus pernio is occassionally the first manifestation of sarcoidosis but it tends to persist for many years. Lupus pernio appears as purple-red swellings, which resemble chilblains, on the nose, cheeks, fingers and toes.

Superficial lymph nodes
Superficial lymphadenopathy occurs in 30 per cent of patients and sometimes lymph nodes in more than one region are enlarged. The cervical, supraclavicular, axillary and epitrochlear nodes are most frequently involved. Sarcoid nodes are small, discrete, firm and nontender. The parotid glands are sometimes enlarged.

Eyes
The eyes are involved in about 30 per cent of patients. Acute uveitis is the commonest ocular manifestation and causes watering, redness and discomfort of the eye and keratic precipitates in the anterior chamber.

Acute uveitis is a manifestation of subacute sarcoidosis and may accompany bilateral hilar lymphadenopathy. Chronic uveitis may cause secondary glaucoma, cataract and blindness. Uveitis, parotid swelling and fever (uveo-parotid fever) accompanied by facial palsy is an unusual manifestation of sarcoidosis.

Liver and spleen
These organs are commonly infiltrated with sarcoid granulomas but the liver is rarely enlarged and the spleen is palpable only 10 per cent of patients.

Uncommon manifestations
Nervous system. Sarcoidosis involves the nervous system in 5 per cent of patients. It may affect the cranial and peripheral nerves. brain, spinal cord and meninges. The commonest manifestations are cranial nerve lesions and peripheral neuropathy. Facial palsy of lower motor neurone type is present in 50 per cent of patients with sarcoidosis of the nervous system. Sarcoid infiltration of the men-

inges and granulomas in the brain may cause meningitis, motor and sensory disturbances, diabetes insipidus, confusion and fits.

Skeletal system. Febrile arthralgia may accompany erythema nodosum or bilateral hilar lymphadenopathy. In chronic sarcoidosis, cysts occasionally develop in the phalanges of the hands and feet. Sarcoid granulomas in muscle may cause myopathy.

Kidneys and calcium metabolism. Sarcoid infiltration of the kidney is uncommon and rarely causes impaired renal function. Hypercalcaemia may occur as a result of increased absorption of calcium from the bowel due to increased sensitivity to vitamin D. Hypercalcaemia and hypercalcuria may cause renal damage leading to renal failure. Calcium deposition in the kidneys, nephrocalcinosis, may be detected radiographically.

Heart. Sarcoid infiltration of the heart may cause heart block and other arrhythmias. Cor pulmonale is a terminal event in patients with extensive pulmonary fibrosis due to chronic sarcoidosis.

INVESTIGATIONS

Chest radiograph. The radiographic appearances of sarcoidosis are shown in Figures 35 and 36. Bilateral hilar lymphadenopathy causes symmetrical, smooth hilar enlargement and sometimes the paratracheal nodes are also enlarged. The lymphadenopathy may be accompanied by pulmonary lesions.

Pulmonary sarcoidosis has a variable radiographic appearance. In the early stages the opacities vary in size from 1 to 5 mm and produce miliary mottling or nodular shadowing. These abnormalities involve most of the lung fields but sometimes the mid zones are pre-

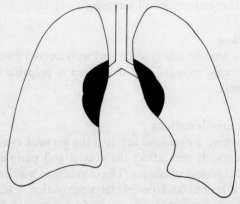

Fig. 35 Sarcoidosis. Bilateral hilar lymphadenopathy showing smooth symmetrical hilar enlargement.

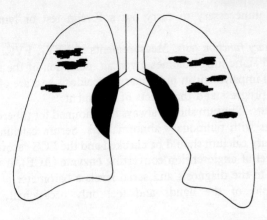

Fig. 36 Sarcoidosis. Bilateral hilar lymphadenopathy with patchy parenchymal lesions.

dominantly affected. Occasionally sarcoidosis causes patchy confluent shadows. Chronic sarcoidosis usually causes dense mid-zone fibrosis with patchy fibrosis elsewhere.

Tuberculin test. About 60 per cent of patients have a negative reaction to 100 TU. With the decline of tuberculosis it may become appropriate to test delayed hypersensitivity with a common allergen such as *C. albicans*.

Kveim test. The Kveim test is positive in 70–80 per cent of patients with sarcoidosis and is more likely to be positive in patients with active disease. An intradermal injection of 0.1 ml of a suspension of human sarcoid tissue is given in the forearm. Within two to three weeks a positive reaction shows a purplish-red nodule at the injection site. The nodule is biopsied 4 to 6 weeks after the injection and shows sarcoid tissue on histological examination. A positive Kveim test is virtually diagnostic of sarcoidosis and false positives are rare if a good Kveim antigen is used. False positives may arise if the Kveim antigen is contaminated during preparation. A positive Kveim test may occur in Crohn's disease but this unlikely to be confused clinically with sarcoidosis. The Kveim reaction is suppressed by corticosteroids and if possible these should not be given until the test is read.

Tissue biopsy. Biopsy of a supraclavicular or epitrochlear lymph node will provide a histological diagnosis in 90 per cent of patients. Biopsy of skin lesions, transbronchial lung biopsy and mediastinoscopy are equally successful.

In many cases, particularly those with hilar lymphadenopathy and erythema nodosum, the diagnosis can be made on clinical grounds, and it is unnecessary to carry out a Kveim test or lymph node biopsy.

Pulmonary function tests. Measurements of FEV_1, FVC, Transfer factor and static lung volumes given an indication of the degree of functional impairment in pulmonary sarcoidosis and are of value in assessing progress and the effects of treatment.

Other tests. Sputum should always be examined for tubercle bacilli in patients with pulmonary abnormalities. Serum calcium and 24 hour urinary calcium should be checked and the ECG recorded. The serum level of angiotension converting enzyme (ACE), if raised, is a pointer to the diagnosis and serial levels a barometer of activity. Radiographs of the hands and feel only occasionally help in diagnosis.

DIFFERENTIAL DIAGNOSIS

Lymphoma; metastatic malignancy. These diseases caused hilar lymphadenopathy, but usually it is unilateral and there is a history of weight loss and ill health which are uncommon features in sarcoidosis.

Erythema nodosum may be a manifestation of primary tuberculosis, streptococcal infection or histoplasmosis, but none of these diseases are likely to cause bilateral hilar lymphadenopathy.

Tuberculosis; pneumoconiosis. Diseases which cause miliary or nodular radiographic abnormalities must be differentiated from pulmonary sarcoidosis. If the patient is well and has no occupational history of dust exposure, sarcoidosis is the most likely diagnosis. In doubtful cases a Kveim test, transbronchial biopsy or lymph node biopsy should be carried out.

Fibrosing alveolitis. Breathlessness is usually more severe than in sarcoidosis and in the majority of cases finger clubbing is present.

TREATMENT

There is no known cure for sarcoidosis but in most cases corticosteroids will suppress the disease. Sarcoidosis frequently resolves spontaneously and treatment with corticosteroids is necessary only when vital organs are involved. There is no indication for corticosteroid therapy in hilar lymphadenopathy.

Corticosteroids are indicated in pulmonary sarcoidosis if there is severe breathlessness or significant impairment of function or radiographic evidence of progression of parenchymal lesions after three months observation or lack of radiological resolution after six months observation. The decision to use corticosteroids is preferably based upon evidence of impaired function than on the radiographic appearances.

Initially prednisolone 20 to 40 mg daily is given and the effects of treatment are assessed clinically and by serial measurements of ventilatory function and transfer factor. When maximum improvement has occurred, the dose of prednisolone is gradually reduced to a level which maintains suppression. The usual maintenance dose is about 10 mg daily. Effective suppression should be maintained for at least 2 years before attempting gradual withdrawal of prednisolone. Corticosteroids are not usually effective in patients with chronic fibrosis.

Corticosteroids are also indicated when sarcoidosis affects the eyes, nervous system or heart, or if hypercalcaemia or hypercalcuria are present. Oxyphenbutazone and chloroquine suppress the manifestations of sarcoidosis but are not as effective as corticosteroids.

Antituberculosis drugs should be given to patients receiving corticosteroids if there is evidence of previous tuberculosis.

COURSE AND PROGNOSIS

Table 20 outlines the course of subacute and chronic sarcoidosis. Usually the disease is self limiting. In 80 per cent of patients the hilar lymphadenopathy resolves spontaneously within one year and in a further 10 per cent resolution occurs in the second year. Pulmonary opacities clear spontaneously within two years in 60 per cent of patients. About 10 per cent develop chronic pulmonary fibrosis which may cause cor pulmonale. Cerebral sarcoidosis may be fatal.

FURTHER READING

Crofton J, Douglas A 1981 Respiratory diseases. 3rd edn. Blackwell, Oxford
Lancet 1972 Kveim-Siltzbach test vindicated. Leading article i:188
Marshall R Karlish A J 1971 Lung function in sarcoidosis. Thorax 26:402
Mitchell D N, Rees R J W 1969 A transmissible agent from sarcoid tissue. Lancet ii:81
Mitchell D N, Scadding J G 1974 Sarcoidosis. American Review of Respiratory Diseases State of the Art. vol 110:774
Scadding J G 1967 Sarcoidosis. Lyre & Spottiswoode, London
Scadding J G 1973 The treatment of sarcoidosis. Prescriber's Journal 12:95

20

Occupational lung diseases

DEFINITION AND CLASSIFICATION

Occupational lung diseases are a group of varied disorders caused by occupational exposure to dusts, gases or fumes. Inhaled particles produce a variety of reactions in the respiratory tract which depend upon the nature of the inhaled matter; the size, shape and concentration of the particles, the degree and duration of exposure, the site of the reaction and the individual worker's susceptibility. Particles of 5 μ or less in diameter may reach the alveoli; larger particles are deposited on the bronchial tree and are expectorated.

Occupational lung diseases may be broadly classified into the following groups:

1. Pneumoconioses. These diseases are caused by prolonged inhalation of *inorganic dusts* which accumulate in the lungs, causing tissue reactions, e.g. coalworkers' pneumoconiosis.

2. Extrinsic allergic alveolitis. This group of diseases is due to inhalation of *organic dusts* which produce a type 3 hyper-sensitivity reaction in the lungs, e.g. farmers' lung.

3. Occupational asthma. Certain dusts and furmes encountered in different occupations predominantly affect the bronchi, causing acute airways obstruction, e.g. toluene diisocyanate asthma.

4. Reactions due to irritant gases and fumes. Inhalation of irritant gases and fumes causes acute bronchial irritation and acute pulmonary oedema, e.g. chlorine.

PNEUMOCONIOSES

The pneumoconioses are named according to the causal dust, and the principal types and the relevant occupations are shown in Table 21. Uncommon causes of pneumoconiosis include barium, iron, tin, aluminium, mica and talc. The pneumoconioses are the commonest occupational lung diseases. Regular supervision of workers in hazardous occupations and constant attention to dust suppression are carried out by government departments of industrial medicine. The differential diagnosis includes diseases which cause diffuse radiographic abnormalities such as tuberculosis, sarcoidosis and fibrosing alveolitis.

Table 21 Principal types of pneumoconiosis

Pneumoconiosis	Causal dust	Occupation
Coalworkers' pneumoconiosis	Coal dust	Coal mining
Silicosis	Silica	Mining, quarrying, stone dressing, sand blasting, pottery industry
Asbestosis	Asbestos	Insulating workers, asbestos manufacture, shipyard workers and dockers.

Coalworkers' pneumoconiosis

Coalworkers' pneumoconiosis is the commonest type of pneumoconiosis and develops in miners who have been exposed to coal dust for several years. The prevalence of coalworkers' pneumoconiosis shows considerable geographic variation which is mainly related to the quality of the coal and the efficiency of the methods of dust suppression.

Coal dust is deposited around the alveoli and respiratory bronchioles where it stimulates focal proliferation of reticulin fibres causing nodular and diffuse fibrosis. Dilatation of the respiratory bronchioles gives rise to focal emphysema. This stage of the disease is known as *simple pneumoconsiosis*. Progressive fibrosis produces dense circumscribed fibrotic masses in the upper lobes which is termed *complicated pneumoconiosis* or *progressive massive fibrosis* (PMF). Sometimes these lesions cavitate with expectoration of black sputum (melanoptysis). The cause of PMF is not known and theories that it is due to tuberculous or atypical mycobacterial infection have not been substantiated.

Simple pneumoconiosis does not usually cause symptoms, but with the development of PMF the miner becomes increasingly breathless and may eventually develop cor pulmonale. Cough and sputum are usually due to chronic bronchitis which is more common in miners than in those employed in other occupations, but is nevertheless thought to be predominantly related to cigarette smoking among miners. Examination of the chest is often normal and finger clubbing is rare.

In simple pneumoconiosis the chest radiograph shows miliary mottling (diffuse opacities 2 mm or less in diameter) or diffuse nodular opacities 3 to 10 mm in diameter. Single or multiple homogeneous opacities greater than 1 cm in diameter indicate the presence of PMF.

Simple coalworkers' pneumoconiosis does not usually progress if further dust exposure is avoided, but PMF usually becomes progressively worse even when the worker is no longer exposed to coal dust. Miners who develop pneumoconiosis are advised to work in areas where dust concentrations are comparatively low unless they have minimal disease. Most governments provide compensation for workers with complicated pneumoconiosis.

Caplan's syndrome. This syndrome comprises pneumoconiosis, rheumatoid arthritis and rheumatoid nodules in the lung. The nodules are single or multiple and occur in the periphery of the lung. These nodules show the histoligical features of rheumatoid arthritis and may appear before, with, or after the clinical onset of the arthritis.

Silicosis
Silica dust has a marked capacity to cause severe fibrosis in the lungs, and in silicosis fibrotic nodules occur diffusely throughout the lungs. Extensive fibrosis gives rise to PMF and cor pulmonale. Generally several years exposure is necessary before silicosis develops. The fibrosis is progressive and the patient may not develop evidence of silicosis until many years after dust exposure has ceased.

Initially there may be no symptoms despite radiographic evidence of silicosis; later the patient develops breathlessness which becomes progressively more severe. Silicosis does not cause finger clubbing. The chest radiograph shows diffuse nodular shadowing and occasionally there is 'egg shell' calcification of the periphery of the hilar lymph nodes.

Workers with silicosis are usually advised to avoid further dust exposure and they are kept under regular surveillance because silicosis predisposes to tuberculosis. Silicosis is compensatable.

Asbestosis
Asbestos is used widely for insulation in ship building, brake and clutch manufacturing, roofing and in the electrical industry. Asbestosis only develops after many years' exposure to asbestos. Asbestos fibres stimulate dense fibrosis in the walls of the bronchioles and alveoli, particularly in the lower lobes. The fibres penetrate to the

pleura and cause dense pleural fibrosis. PMF does not occur in asbestosis. Asbestosis is compensatable.

The main functional abnormality is reduction in transfer factor, although severe fibrosis gives rise to the characteristic findings of restrictive lung disease. Frequently there are no symptoms but severe fibrosis causes breathlessness, cough, central cyanosis and bilateral lower lobe crepitations. Finger clubbing is common. The chest radiograph is normal or shows streaky reticular shadowing predominantly in the lower zones where it may obscure the outline of the heart and diaphragm. Pleural thickening is common. Asbestos bodies can be demonstrated in sputum smears and indicate exposure to asbestos, but they do not signify asbestosis for they are sometimes present in the sputum and lungs of healthy people. An asbestos body consists of an asbestos fibre covered with a film of protein impregnated with iron and for this reason is sometimes called 'a ferruginous body'.

There is no specific treatment and the value of corticosteroids is doubtful. The patient should avoid further exposure to asbestos.

Other manifestations of asbestos exposure

Bronchial carcinoma. Incidence is increased in people with asbestosis. Cigarette smoking interacts synergistically with asbestosis towards lung cancer risk.

Pleural plaques. Asbestos causes plaques of fibrosis and calcification on the pleura. These do not give rise to symptoms but cause calcification in the chest radiograph which is often bilateral and mainly occurs in the lower half of the thorax. Calcification in the diaphragmatic pleura is pathognomic of asbestos exposure.

Pleural and peritoneal mesothelioma. Exposure to blue asbestos may cause diffuse mesothelioma of the pleura or peritoneum after a latent period of 20 years. Sometimes the exposure has been transient and minimal. Pleural mesothelioma may present with chest pain, or breathlessness secondary to pleural effusion or as a chance radiological finding. The effusion is usually bloodstained. Diagnosis can be confirmed by pleural biopsy if the occupational history, clinical and radiological findings are not conclusive. There is no curative treatment which therefore is purely palliative. Death usually ensues in less than two years from diagnosis. Mesothelioma is compensatable.

EXTRINSIC ALLERGIC ALVEOLITIS

Definition
Extrinsic allergic alveolitis is a characteristic form of pulmonary

hypersensitivity caused by inhalation of a variety of organic dusts. The pathogenesis, the functional abnormality and the clinical and radiographic features are similar in all types of allergic alveolitis.

Aetiology and pathogenesis

The main types of allergic alveolitis are shown in Table 22 which illustrates the varied situations which predispose to allergic alveolitis and the importance of occupational exposure. In most types the causal antigens are thermophilic fungi which proliferate in organic matter under conditions of high humidity and temperate. Allergic alveolitis is uncommon except for farmer's lung, which occurs after working with hay which has been harvested while damp and then stored in barns.

Table 22 Main types of extrinsic allergic alveolitis

Allergic alveolitis	Causal agent	Antigen
Farmer's lung	Mouldy hay	*Micropolyspora faeni* *Thermoactinomyces vulgaris*
Bird fancier's lung	Pigeon, budgerigar droppings	Serum protein and droppings
Bagassosis	Mouldy sugar cane bagasse	*T. vulgaris*
Pituitary snuff taker's lung	Heterologous pituitary powder used to treat diabetes insipidus	Serum protein and pituitary extracts
Malt worker's lung	Mouldy barley, malt	*Aspergillus clavatus*
Mushroom worker's lung	Mushroom compost	*M. faenit, T. vulgaris*
Humidifier fever	Humidifier water	Cephalosporium? Amoebae?

Allergic alveolitis develops predominantly in non-atopic individuals who may become sensitized to organic dusts as a result of repeated exposure. Further exposure to the dust causes an attack of allergic alveolitis which is a type 3 precipitin-mediated hypersensitivity reaction. An antigen-antibody reaction occurs in the alveolar walls and symptoms develop 4 to 6 hours after exposure. The alveolar reaction is accompanied by systemic and pulmonary symptoms.

Exposure to high concentrations of antigen causes acute allergic alveolitis whilst repeated exposure to smaller amounts of dust is more likely to lead to subacute or chronic disease. The disease does not become chronic if repeated exposure is avoided.

Pathology and functional abnormality

Histological examination shows thickening of the alveolar walls and interstitium of the lung by oedema, plasma cells, lymphocytes, and epithelioid granulomata. The respiratory bronchioles may also be affected. In chronic cases there is diffuse intestitial fibrosis similar to that seen in fibrosing alveolitis.

The diffuse involvement of the alveolar walls and interstitial tissues gives rise to a restrictive ventilatory abnormality and reduction in diffusing capacity, total lung capacity and pulmonary compliance. Ventilation-perfusion imbalance and impaired gas transfer may cause hypoxaemia and the P_aCO_2 may fall as a result of compensatory hyperventilation.

Clinical features

Onset. The onset is usually acute and symptoms develop 4 to 6 hours after exposure to the causal dust.

Pulmonary symptoms. Breathlessness and unproductive cough are common and are produced by the alveolar reaction. Wheeze is not a dominant symptom.

Systemic symptoms. Fever, shivering, malaise, headache and anorexia accompany the pulmonary symptoms. Weight loss may occur during a severe attack.

Physical examination. Bilateral mid and upper zone crepitations which are 'dry' and crackling in quality are characteristic of allergic alveolitis. Occasionally the patient is extremely ill with severe dyspnoea and central cyanosis. Clubbing of the fingers is rare.

Symptoms subside within days or weeks of cessation of dust exposure, although repeated exposure causes recurrent attacks leading to subacute and chronic forms of the disease, with increasing respiratory disability and cor pulmonale.

Investigations

Chest radiograph. During an attack the chest radiograph may be normal but usually there is fine mottling which produces a ground glass appearance. The abnormalities clear after several weeks but occasionally nodular shadows persist. In chronic cases there is diffuse pulmonary fibrosis with reticular shadowing and cystic changes similar to those seen in fibrosing alveolitis.

Peripheral blood. Slight leucocytosis may occur but eosinophilia is uncommon. ESR rises in the acute stage.

Serological tests. Precipitins against the causal antigen can be detected by double diffusion in most forms of allergic alveolitis. The presence of antibodies against a particular allergen is evidence of previous dust exposure but is not diagnostic of allergic alveolitis because healthy persons may have antibodies. A positive precipitin test in association with the typical clinical features is diagnostic.

Pulmonary function tests. Ventilation tests show a proportionate reduction in both FEV_1 and FVC with a normal FEV_1/FVC ratio. The transfer factor is often severely reduced. Hypoxaemia may be present at rest but in mild cases will appear only after exercise; the P_aCO_2 is normal or low. Ventilation tests and transfer factor are helpful in assessing the course of the disease and the results of treatment.

Bronchial challenge. A causal relationship between an organic dust and allergic alveolitis is confirmed if inhalation tests with the dust provoke the typical symptoms and changes in pulmonary function. Inhalation tests should be carried out with caution since they may provoke a severe reaction and they are usually unnecessary for diagnosis.

Differential diagnosis

Allergic alveolitis should be suspected in any patient with a relevant occupation who suffers recurrent attacks of breathlessness, cough and fever. The delay between exposure and the onset of symptoms is the most helpful diagnostic clue but may be overlooked unless a careful history is taken.

Asthma. In asthma the predominant symptom is wheeze, and in allergic cases symptoms occur immediately after dust exposure. Systemic symptoms are minimal, rhonchi are present and eosinophilia is common. The chest radiograph is normal and there is an obstructive ventilatory abnormality which is reversed by bronchodilators.

Acute bronchitis. Purulent sputum, rhonchi, a normal chest radiograph and response to antibiotics are features of acute bronchitis but not of allergic alveolitis.

Bronchopneumonia. This causes systemic symptoms, cough and breathlessness, but the symptoms often follow an upper respiratory tract infection and the cough is productive of purulent sputum.

Sarcoidosis. The nodular radiographic abnormalities of sarcoidosis may resemble allergic alveolitis, but sarcoidosis does not cause acute attacks of breathlessness, cough and fever.

Fibrosing alveolitis. In fibrosing alveolitis the breathlessness usually begins insidiously and becomes progressively worse; clubbing is common.

Allergic bronchopulmonary aspergillosis. This causes wheeze, migratory pulmonary infiltrations and eosinophilia (p. 119).

Treatment

Treatment is usually unnecessary, but oxygen and prednisolone, 20 to 40 mg daily, are given if the patient is severely ill. The dose of prednisolone is reduced gradually after 1 to 2 weeks; if it is stopped abruptly symptoms may recur. Occasionally corticosteroids are necessary for longer periods, and after a severe attack pulmonary function tests may take many months to return to normal. Bronchodilators and antibiotics are ineffective.

Prevention

Further attacks of allergic alveolitis can be prevented if the patient avoids exposure to the causal antigen. This may be difficult in farmer's lung but can usually be achieved if the patient delegates the job of working with mouldy hay and if hay is dried before storage. A respirator should be worn if contact cannot be avoided. In Britain a patient with farmer's lung may claim compensation under the Industrial Injuries Act.

OCCUPATIONAL ASTHMA

Dust and fumes encountered in different occupations may cause asthma. The mechanisms responsible are not fully understood but some probably represent a combination of type 1 and type 3 hypersensitivity reactions. There is usually a preliminary period of symptomless exposure ranging from days to years. Symptoms of wheezing, tightness of chest, cough and breathlessness usually occur towards the end of the working day or during the night and characteristically the patient does not have symptoms during the weekend or on holiday.

Skin tests help in the diagnosis of sensitivity to platinum salts, proteolytic enzymes and laboratory animals. Bronchial challenge tests are helpful in diagnosis and may produce both an immediate and a late bronchial reaction, with airways obstruction occurring immediately and again 4 to 6 hours after the test. This is called a dual reaction.

Cedar dust asthma. Carpenters and mill workers exposed to the dust of Canadian or Western red cedar may suffer attacks of rhinorrhoea, sneezing, coughing and wheezing. Symptoms mainly occur 4 to 6 hours after exposure.

Proteolytic enzyme washing powders. Workers concerned with the manufacture of enzyme-containing washing powders may develop wheeze, cough and rhinorrhoea after inhalation of enzymes of *Bacillus subtilis* used in their manufacture.

Toluene di-isocyanate. Workers in the plastics, paints and adhesives industries may become sensitized to di-isocyanate and suffer acute wheezing attacks after exposure. Subsequently even tiny quantities of TDI can precipitate an attack. A change of workplace is usually necessary. Asthma may persist even if no further exposure occurs.

Epoxy resins (adhesive, moulding resin, plastic industries), *platinum salts* (platinum refining, laboratories) *colophony* (solder flux), *flour and grain dusts* and *animal and insects in laboratories* are other recognised and compensatable forms of occupational asthma.

Byssinosis. Workers in the cotton and flax industry may become hypersensitive to cotton dust and develop acute wheeze when the return to work on Monday. Recurrent exposure causes chronic wheeze and breathlessness. The condition is accepted as a compensatable industrial pulmonary disease.

REACTIONS TO IRRITANT GASES AND FUMES

Irritant gases such as ammonia, chlorine, phosgene, sulphur dioxide and nitrogen dioxide can cause acute inflammation of the eyes and respiratory tract. Coughing, breathlessness and a choking sensation occur immediately after exposure, and acute pulmonary oedema may develop after an interval of several hours. Occasionally permanent bronchial damage results in chronic cough, sputum and breathlessness. Fumes of metals or their inorganic compounds, such as nickel, platinum, vanadium and tungsten cause acute bronchial irritation resulting in attacks of coughing and wheezing. Severe reactions to gases and fumes may require treatment with corticosteroids and oxygen.

FURTHER READING

Chan-Yeung M, Barton G M, Maclean L, Grzybowski S 1973 Occupational asthma and rhinitis due to Western red cedar (Thuja plicata). American Review of Respiratory Diseases 108:1094

Channell S, Blyth W, Lloyd M, Weir D M, Amos W M G, Littlewood A P, Riddle H F V, Grant I W B 1969 Allergic alveolitis in maltworkers: a clinical, mycological and immunological study. Quarterly Journal of Medicine 18:351

Cockroft A, Edwards J, Bevan C, Campbell I, Collins G, Houston K, Jenkins D, Latham S, Saunders M, Trotman D 1981 An investigation of operating theatre staff exposed to humidifier fever antigens. British Journal of Industrial Medicine, 38:144

Dijkman J H, Borghans J G A, Savelberg P J, Arkenbout P M 1973 Allergic bronchial reactions to inhalation of enzymes of Bacillus subtilis. American Review of Respiratory Diseases 107:387

Hapke E J, Seal R M E, Thomas G O, Hayes M, Meek J C 1969 Farmer's lung: A clinical, radiographic, functional, and seriological correlation of acute and chronic stages. Thorax 23:451

Hargreave F E, Pepys J Longbottom J L Wraith D G 1966 Bird breeder's (fancier's) lung. Lancet i:445

Hargreave F E, Pepys J, Holford-Strevens V 1968 Bagassosis. Lancet i:619

HMSO 1982 Clinical notes on occupational asthma. D.H.S.S. Ref. NI 238/March 1982

Hunter D 1978 The diseases of occupations. 6th ed. English Universities Press, London

Morgan W K C, Seaton A 1975 Occupational lung disease. Saunders, Philadelphia

Ryder R, Lyons J P, Campbell H, Gough J 1970 Emphysema in coal worker's pneumoconiosis. British Medical Journal iii:481

21

Pulmonary fibrosis and diffuse fibrosing alveolitis

Pulmonary fibrosis may complicate almost any type of pulmonary disease and forms part of the local response to injury whatever the cause.

There are three main types of pulmonary fibrosis: *1. Replacement fibrosis*. This form of fibrosis follows diseases which damage the lung parenchyma, such as pneumonia, tuberculosis and bronchiectasis. It is usually not sufficiently extensive to cause symptoms but when it is predominantly unilateral it may produce the signs of localized pulmonary fibrosis, e.g. reduced movement of the chest wall, mediastinal displacement, reduced percussion note and decreased breath sounds (p. 41).

2. Focal fibrosis. Focal fibrosis forms part of the tissue reaction to inhalation of inorganic dust and is a feature of pneumoconiosis.

3. Interstitial fibrosis. Fibrosis may predominantly involve the interstitial tissue of the lung in diseases such as sarcoidosis, extrinsic allergic alveolitis, and diffuse fibrosing alveolitis.

Pulmonary fibrosis is essentially a pathological term and the different forms of fibrosis do not give rise to a single clinical entity. It is perferable to consider pulmonary fibrosis in relation to the different diseases which produce it.

DIFFUSE FIBROSING ALVEOLITIS

Definition
Diffuse fibrosing alveolitis is the term proposed by Scadding to describe inflammation in the lung beyond the terminal bronchiole, having two essential histological features:
1. Cellular thickening of the alveolar walls showing a tendency to fibrosis (mural).
2. The presence of large mononuclear cells presumably of alveolar origin within the air spaces (desquamative).

Although this definition is based on the pathological findings, fibrosing alveolitis causes characteristic physiological abnormalities and distinctive clinical and radiographic features.

The earliest description was made by Hamman and Rich and referred to an acute fatal type of interstitial fibrosis, the *Hamman-Rich syndrome*. Chronic forms of the disease have been termed *diffuse interstitial pulmonary fibrosis*. The term *desquamative interstitial pneumonia* has been given to cases in which the predominant finding is extensive alveolar cell proliferation and desquamation, equivalent to Scadding's desquamative fibrosing alveolitis. Response to corticosteroids is more likely in the desquamative form than in the mural form of fibrosing alveolitis.

Epidemiology
Fibrosing alveolitis is an uncommon disorder and occurs mainly in those over the age of 40; the sex distribution is equal.

Aetiology
Cryptogenic fibrosing alveolitis. In the majority of cases of fibrosing alveolitis there is no history of exposure to any known aetiological agent and there is no clinical evidence of diseases known to be associated with fibrosing alveolitis.

Collagen disorders. Fibrosing alveolitis is sometimes found in patients with collagen disorders; it occurs in 5 per cent of patients with rheumatoid arthritis and in 30 per cent of patients with systemic sclerosis. Fibrosing alveolitis is occasionally associated with systemic lupus erythematosus and chronic active hepatitis.

Drugs. Fibrosing alveolitis is a rare complication of treatment with hexamethonium, busulphan and chlorambucil.

Pathology and functional abnormality
The earliest histological findings are the accumulation of large mononuclear cells and fibrinous exudate in the alveoli and slight cellular thickening of the alveolar walls. At this stage progression of the disease may be prevented by corticosteroids. Later there is marked interstitial fibrosis with fibrotic thickening of the alveolar walls, which is unlikely to be affected by corticosteroids. With increasing fibrosis the lungs become small and stiff and the normal architecture may be replaced by small cysts. The diffuse interstitial abnormalities produce a restrictive ventilatory defect and reduction in total lung capacity, pulmonary compliance and diffusing capacity. Ventilation-perfusion imbalance and impaired gas transfer result in hypoxaemia especially on exercise. The patient compensates by hyperventilation which may cause hypocapnia.

Clinical features

Fibrosing alveolitis may be acute or chronic. In the rare acute form symptoms begin suddenly and the course of the illness is rapid.

Breathlessness. This is the commonest presenting symptom and in the chronic form the onset is insidious. Characteristically the dyspnoea becomes progressively more severe. Wheeze is not a feature of fibrosing alveolitis.

Cough. Cough is common and initially it is unproductive, but later purulent sputum may be expectorated as a result of secondary bacterial infection.

Weight loss and fatigue. These are common features in the acute form and in the later stages of the chronic form. Fever is sometimes a feature of acute fibrosing alveolitis.

Physical examination. Clubbing of the fingers occurs in 80 per cent of patients. Central cyanosis may be present, especially after exercise. Respiration is rapid and shallow and the chest expansion is decreased. On auscultation the characteristic finding is dry crackling crepitations over both lower lobes.

Early in the disease there may be no symptoms and signs and it is only detected on routine radiography. Arthritis and systemic signs are present when fibrosing alveolitis is a manifestation of a collagen disorder, although arthopathy sometimes occurs in the absence of collagen disorder.

Investigations

Chest radiograph. Initially the chest radiograph may be normal despite the presence of symptoms. In the acute form there may be patchy shadows resembling bronchopneumonia. More commonly, fibrosing alveolitis causes bilateral miliary or nodular shadows 1 to 5 mm in diameter and/or streaky reticular opacities (Fig. 37). These abnormalities are most marked in the lower zones and in the later stages small cystic translucencies produce a honeycomb appearance. Shrinkage of the lungs causes elevation of the diaphragm.

Pulmonary function tests. The main abnormalities are marked reduction in FVC and TLCO. The total lung capacity and pulmonary compliance are also reduced and eventually blood gas analysis shows hypoxaemia and hypocapnia.

Peripheral blood. Secondary polycythaemia may occur in the chronic form of the disease. The ESR is sometimes raised.

Immunological studies. In 30 per cent of patients without clinical evidence of collagen disorders the serum globulins are increased and rheumatoid factor and antinuclear factor are present. Non-organ specific antibodies are also present in 30 per cent of patients.

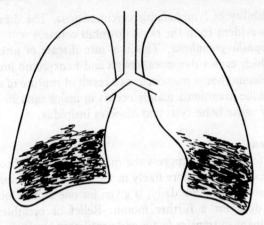

Fig. 37 Fibrosing alveolitis. Reticular shadowing in both mid and lower zones.

Lung biopsy. Usually it is possible to make the diagnosis on clinical and radiographic grounds. Lung biopsy may be necessary in doubtful cases or to assess the probability of response to corticosteroids.

Differential diagnosis

Bronchopneumonia. Pneumonia must be considered in the differential diagnosis of the acute form of fibrosing alveolitis. The symptoms and signs of bronchopneumonia resolve rapidly after antibiotic therapy.

Pulmonary oedema. This can be differentiated from fibrosing alveolitis by the presence of cardiomegaly and the rapid disappearance of dyspnoea and crepitations after diuretic therapy.

Allergic alveolitis. This causes transient respiratory and systemic symptoms 4 to 6 hours after exposure to the causal organic dust. Finger clubbing is rare in allergic alveolitis. Precipitins to the causal antigen can often be demonstrated. It may be impossible to differentiate the chronic form of allergic alveolitis from fibrosing alveolitis.

Sarcoidosis. Finger clubbing is rare in pulmonary sarcoidosis, and breathlessness is less severe than in fibrosing alveolitis. There may be clinical evidence of sarcoidosis elsewhere, and the Kveim test or tissue biopsy confirms the diagnosis.

Asbestosis. This may resemble fibrosing alveolitis radiographically and should be suspected if there is an occupational history of exposure to asbestos.

Lymphangitis carcinomatosa. Progressive breathlessness, weight loss, malaise and bilateral streaky radiographic abnormalities suggest the possibility of lymphangitis carcinomatosa. The diagnosis soon becomes evident from the rapid downhill course.

Eosinophilic granuloma. This is a rare disease of unknown aetiology which causes dyspnoea, cough and honeycomb lung. Spontaneous pneumothorax may occur as a result of rupture of a lung cyst. Eosinophilic granuloma mainly occurs in males aged 20 to 40 years and may cause bone cysts and diabetes insipidus.

Treatment

Corticosteroids may suppress the manifestations of fibrosing alveolitis, response being more likely in the desquamative sort.

Prednisolone, 40 mg daily, is given for one month followed by a smaller dose for a further month. Relief of breathlessness and improvement in transfer factor and ventilatory levels are indications for long-term treatment with prednisolone, the dose gradually being reduced to the lowest level that will control the disease. Azathioprine may permit some sparing of corticosteroid dosage.

In the mural type or chronic form of fibrosing alveolitis corticosteroids are usually ineffective and treatment is directed towards control of respiratory infections, heart failure and respiratory failure.

Prognosis

Most patients die from respiratory failure and cor pulmonale within four years but a good response to corticosteroids improves the prognosis. In the acute form, if there is no response, death occurs within six months.

FUTHER READING

Johnson A J 1982 Cryptogenic fibrosing alveolitis. Hospital Update Sept:1085

Johnson A J, Honey R M, Turner-Warwick M, Hinson K F W 1977 Corticosteroid treatment and the prognosis of cryptogenic fibrosing alveolitis. Thorax 32:650

Scadding J G 1964 Fibrosing alveolitis. British Medical Journal ii:686

Scadding J G 1970 Lung biopsy in the diagnosis of diffuse lung disease. British Medical Journal ii:557

Scadding J G, Hinson K F W 1967 Diffuse fibrosing alveolitis (diffuse interstitial fibrosis of the lungs): correlation of histology at biopsy with prognosis. Thorax 22:291

Stack B H R 1971 The clinical manifestations and diagnosis of fibrosing alveolitis. British Thoracic and Tuberculosis Association Review 1:15

Turner-Warwick M, Haslam P 1971 Antibodies in some chronic fibrosing lung diseases. Clinical Allergy 1:83

22

Pleural effusion

DEFINITION

Pleural effusion is the term applied to a collection of fluid in the pleural space which results from transudation or exudation. It is not generally applied to a collection of blood (haemothorax, p. 234), chyle (chylothorax, p. 234) or pus (empyema, p. 97), although often this differentiation is possible only after the fluid has been aspirated.

AETIOLOGY AND PATHOGENESIS

The visceral and parietal layers of the pleura are normally separated by a thin film of fluid. Fluid passes outwards from the subpleural capillaries into the pleural space and is absorbed by the pleural lymphatics. The following factors are related to the development of pleural effusion:

1. Increased pulmonary capillary pressure.
2. Increased pleural capillary permeability.
3. Decreased pleural lymphatic absorption.
4. Decreased plasma osmotic pressure.
5. Sodium retention.

The diseases which cause pleural effusion are summarized in Table 23. Congestive heart failure and malignancy are the commonest causes.

Pleural effusions may be transudates or exudates.

Transudates result from the passive transudation of fluid into the pleural space and the pleura itself is not involved by disease. The presence of a transudate in the pleural space is termed *hydrothorax*. Transudation occurs if the pulmonary capillary pressure is increased as in congestive heart failure or if there is hypoproteinaemia, e.g.

Table 23 Causes of pleural effusion

Common
Congestive heart failure
Malignancy*: bronchial carcinoma
metastatic carcinoma
Pulmonary infarction*
Less common
Pneumonia*
Tuberculosis*
Collagen disorders*: rheumatoid arthritis
systemic lupus erythematosus
Rare
Nephrotic syndrome
Cirrhosis
Myxoedema
Meigs' syndrome = pleural effusion, ascites, benign ovarian tumour.

*In these diseases the effusion is an exudate.

nephrosis, cirrhosis. The cause of transudation in myxoedema and Meigs' syndrome is not known.

Exudates are secondary to involvement of the pleura by malignancy or inflammation and are due to impaired lymphatic absorption or increased capillary permeability.

Transudates are differentiated from exudates by the protein content and the specific gravity of the pleural fluid. Transudates have a protein content of less than 3 g/100 ml and a specific gravity of less than 1.015. Exudates have a higher protein content and specific gravity than transudates due to protein leakage into the pleural space and decreased lymphatic absorption. Because of the high protein content exudates are often yellow or amber in colour and clot immediately after aspiration.

Usually the fluid collects in the lower part of the pleural space where it compresses the lung, causing reduction in lung volume and restriction of ventilation. Large effusions displace the mediastinum to the opposite side. Sometimes the fluid is localized by pulmonary adhesions (*loculated or encysted effusion*) or collects in the fissures between the lobes of the lung (*interlobar effusion*). Rarely an effusion develops between the lung and the diaphragm (*infrapulmonary effusion*).

CLINICAL FEATURES

Breathlessness. This is the dominant symptom of pleural effusion. The degree of breathlessness depends upon the size of the effusion and the patient's respiratory function. Even small effusions cause dyspnoea in patients with severe impairment of function due to diseases such as chronic bronchitis.

Pleuritic pain. Effusion secondary to disease of the pleura is commonly preceded by pleuritic pain, which occurs at the site of the pleural involvement but may be referred to the shoulder if the central diaphragmatic pleura is affected.

The other symptoms associated with effusion depend on the cause, and the clinical features peculiar to different types of effusion will be discussed separately.

Physical examination. There may be no abnormal findings if the effusion is small. Large effusions cause reduced movement of the chest wall, displacement of the mediastinum to the opposite side, decreased vocal fremitus, dullness on percussion and diminished breath sounds and vocal resonance. Sometimes bronchial breathing is heard over the upper border of an effusion.

The characteristic sign of pleural effusion is stony dullness on percussion, and, since most effusions involve the general pleural space, the dullness extends in a semicircle from the front to the back of the chest. There is also marked resistance to percussion.

INVESTIGATIONS

The diagnosis of pleural effusion must first be confirmed and then the cause determined.

Chest radiograph. The radiographic appearance of a pleural effusion is characteristic. A small effusion causes obliteration of the costophrenic angle and sometimes a thin layer of fluid extends up the lateral chest wall. Large effusions cause a dense homogeneous opacity which occupies the lower part of the hemithorax and is continuous with the radiographic density produced by the diaphragm and mediastinum. The upper border of the opacity is concave and extends laterally to reach its highest point in the axilla. A massive effusion obliterates most or all of the lung field and causes mediastinal displacement to the opposite side (Fig. 38). After pleural aspiration the chest radiograph may show pulmonary abnormalities which had previously been obscured by the effusion.

A loculated effusion causes a semicircular opacity which lies on the lateral chest wall or in the paravertebral gutter. An interlobar effusion causes a localized elliptical opacity which lies along one of the fissures of the lung. An infrapulmonary effusion has an appearance similar to that caused by elevation of the hemidiaphragm. Occasionally it is necessary to take a radiograph in the lateral decubitus position to demonstrate the presence of a small effusion. The

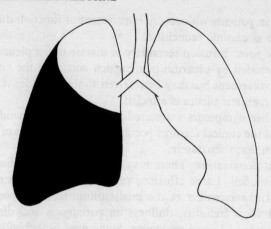

Fig. 38 Pleural effusion showing a homogeneous opacity with a curved upper border and mediastinal displacement to the opposite side.

fluid then tracks up the lateral chest wall unless prevented by adhesions.

Pleural aspiration. This is essential if the cause of the effusion is not known, because examination of the fluid may reveal the diagnosis. Before aspiration it is important to check whether the effusion is on the right or left; it is not unknown for aspiration to have been attempted on the wrong side. The needle is inserted in the midscapular line, one interspace below the point of maximal dullness, and is directed towards the lower part of the interspace to avoid damage to the large intercostal vessels. Aspiration of small effusions is facilitated if a continuous pull is applied to the plunger of the syringe just as the needle is inserted through the parietal pleura. This results in prompt return of fluid and avoids passing the needle beyond the pleural space into the lung. If the latter occurs frothy blood is aspirated. A loculated effusion rarely requires aspiration.

During aspiration care must be taken to prevent air entering the pleural space and the needle must be kept firmly attached to the syringe. It is advisable to limit the quantity of fluid removed on any one occasion to 1500 ml. Aspiration of larger amounts may precipitate unilateral pulmonary oedema.

The colour of the fluid is noted and at least 50 ml is collected for examination for protein, specific gravity, glucose and cells including malignant cells. The specimen for cell is collected in a bottle containing citrate to prevent clotting. Specimens are sent for bacteriological examination, including smear and culture for *M. tuberculosis*.

Table 24 outlines the different characteristics of pleural fluid and their aetiological significance. These characteristics only provide a guide to the possible cause of the effusion and are not diagnostic unless malignant cells or tubercle bacilli are found.

Pleural biopsy. This should be carried out at the time of the aspiration unless the cause of the effusion is known. The Abrams pleural biopsy punch is used and provides a histological diagnosis in 60 per cent of effusion due to malignancy or tuberculosis. Pleural biopsy should not be attempted in the absence of effusion because it may damage the lung.

Further investigations are determined by the history, the clinical findings and the results of pleural aspiration and biopsy. Investigations should always include a tuberculin test and sputum examination for *M. tuberculosis* and malignant cells.

Table 24 The characteristics of pleural fluid related to the possible cause.

	Characteristics	Cause
Colour	clear	Transudate
	amber or yellow	Exudate
	blood stained	Malignancy, pulmonary infarction
	blood	Haemothorax
	milky	Chylothorax
	pus	Empyema
Protein content	< 3 g%	Transudate
	> 3 g%	Exudate
Specific gravity	<1.015	Transudate
	>1.015	Exuadte
Glucose content	<25 mg%	Collagen disorders, tuberculosis
Cell type	polymorphs	Pneumonia
	lymphocytes	Tuberculosis
	malignant cells	Malignancy
Bacteria		Pneumonia, tuberculosis, empyema.

CLINICAL FEATURES AND TREATMENT OF DIFFERENT TYPES OF PLEURAL EFFUSION

Congestive heart failure — Small R > L + Cardiomegaly,

Pleural effusion is a common complication of severe congestive heart failure and sometimes occurs in association with acute pulmonary oedema. The effusion is usually relatively small and occurs most commonly on the right side but may be bilateral. The patient gives a history of progressive exertional dyspnoea and the signs of heart failure are present. The chest radiograph shows cardiomegaly. The effusion resolves rapidly after diuretic therapy and does not require aspiration.

Malignant pleural effusion

1° bronchial commonly. Mesothelioma
2° rarer. breast or bowel

The commonest cause of malignant pleural effusion is *bronchial carcinoma* (p. 168). Pleural effusion complicates bronchial carcinoma in 10 per cent of cases. It should be suspected in middle-aged males who are heavy smokers, particularly if finger clubbing is present or if there is a history of cough, haemoptysis, and ill health.

Pleural effusion secondary to *metastatic carcinoma* is less common than effusion due to bronchial carcinoma. The primary tumour is commonly situated in the breast or bowel. There may be a history of previous malignancy. A search for the primary tumour should only be undertaken if pleural cytology or histology indicate that chemotherapy might be helpful. In females the breasts and pelvis should always be examined carefully. Lymphangitis carcinomatosa and lymphoma are rare causes of pleural effusion; in both cases the effusion may be bilateral.

Pleural effusion is a common presenting manifestation of *pleural mesothelioma*. This rare tumour occurs predominantly in men who have worked with blue asbestos and there is a latent interval of 20 to 30 years between the time of initial exposure and the development of mesothelioma.

Malig cells in cruckate. or in pleural Bφ.

Malignant effusions reaccumulate rapidly after aspiration and this feature is of diagnostic value. The fluid is often blood-stained.

The diagnosis is established by finding malignant cells in the pleural fluid or neoplastic tissue in the pleural biopsy. Malignant cells may be present in the sputum. If these investigations do not confirm the diagnosis bronchoscopy should be carried out.

Nitrogen mustard 20 mg or tetracycline, 500 mg, injected into the pleural cavity after aspiration, causes pleural adhesions and prevents reaccumulation of fluid in around 50% of patients. The patient is sedated before the injection to prevent pain and nausea. Oral prednisolone may also delay the reaccumulation of malignant effusion but neither treatment is curative. Talc pleurodesis is usually effective and should be considered in recurrent malignant effusions. The prognosis is poor and the patient is usually dead within a year.

Pulmonary infarction — *Small*

This is commonly accompanied by exudation of small amounts of fluid into the pleural space. This is usually only sufficient to cause obliteration of the costophrenic angle. A diagnosis of pulmonary infarction should be considered if there is a predisposing cause or if there has been pleuritic pain, breathlessness and haemoptysis (p. 157). The fluid may be blood-stained or amber but aspiration should rarely be necessary. Anticoagulants are given.

Postpneumonic effusion

Effusion secondary to bacterial pneumonia should be suspected if there is a history of a recent respiratory infection. The development of effusion is often preceded by pleuritic pain and fever. Pleural effusion occurs in 5 per cent of all pneumonias.

Postpneumonic effusions are usually small, and since most pneumonias are treated promptly with antibiotics, the fluid is amber or yellow in colour and sterile on culture. If antibiotic treatment has been delayed, pus may accumulate in the pleural cavity. The predominant cell type is the polymorph. The fluid should be aspirated promptly and a specimen sent for bacteriological examination. Antibiotics, usually penicillin or ampicillin, are given for several weeks. Postpneumonic effusions do not reaccumulate after aspiration and appropriate antibiotic treatment.

Tuberculous pleural effusion   — TB evidence in fluid 60% only in 60% ie often are unstanted

This is now relatively uncommon in Western countries but should be considered when effusion occurs in late childhood, adolescence or old age. A family history of tuberculosis is highly significant unless the child has had BCG, and it is essential that the patient is specifically questioned about these facts. Tuberculous effusion is not confined to early life and may develop at any age; it is sometimes a manifestation of miliary tuberculosis in adults.

In childhood the illness is relatively acute, and pleuritic pain, breathlessness and fever are the presenting symptoms. In adults there may be a history of malaise, night sweats and weight loss. The tuberculin test is strongly positive.

M. tuberculosis is isolated from pleural fluid in only 60 per cent of patients and pleural biopsy provides a diagnosis in a similar proportion. For these reasons the diagnosis of tuberculous pleural effusion is often made on circumstantial evidence, i.e. a contact history of tuberculosis, pleural fluid in which lymphocytes are the predominant cell type and a strongly positive tuberculin test. In such cases it is wise to assume a tuberculous aetiology and give antituberculosis treatment. The methods and principles of treatment are the same as for pulmonary tuberculosis. The pleural cavity is aspirated to dryness. Corticosteroids hasten the resolution of tuberculous pleural effusion but should never be given without antituberculosis drugs. Following treatment the radiograph returns to normal, although there may be residual pleural thickening and calcification.

Collagen disorders — RA. Ex, usually under. talc, Rh factor +ve

Pleural effusion, sometimes bilateral, is an occasional manifestation of collagen disorders. It may complicate any ot these disorders but is most common in rheumatoid arthritis and systemic lupus erythematosus. Other signs of these diseases are invariably present and the pleural fluid often has a low glucose contents. Rheumatoid factor, ANF or LE cells may be found in the fluid. The effusion usually resolves spontaneously.

The nephrotic syndrome, cirrhosis and myxoedema are rare causes of effusion but should be suspected when there is evidence of these diseases. Meigs' syndrome is rare; the syndrome comprises pleural effusion, ascites and a benign ovarian tumour.

Bilateral pleural effusions may complicate cardiac failure and sometimes occur in collagen disorders, miliary tuberculosis, lymphangitis carcinomatosa and lymphoma.

HAEMOTHORAX

Haemothorax is usually the result of severe chest trauma or ruptured aortic aneurysm but may complicate pneumothorax due to rupture of a pleural adhesion containing a blood vessel. The signs of fluid in the pleural space may be overshadowed by the signs of shock. The diagnosis is confirmed by pleural aspiration; thoracotomy may be necessary to locate and stop the bleeding.

CHYLOTHORAX

Chyle may accumulate in the pleural space after rupture of the thoracic duct or a large lymphatic channel. The commonest causes of chylothorax are surgical trauma and chest injury. Chylothorax may develop if carcinoma or lymphoma involves the thoracic duct. The pleural fluid is milky in appearance due to the high fat content, and after standing a layer of fat forms on the surface of the fluid. The milky colour clears if ether is added to the fluid. The fat globules stain with sudan III dye. The diagnosis is confirmed by giving the patient a lipophilic dye to eat; if sudan III is given the pleural fluid becomes red. Lipoprotein electrophoresis of chyle shows chylomicrons. Milky effusions which do not contain chylomicrons and do not take up dye are not due to chylothorax.

Chylothorax causes loss of large amounts of protein and is treated by injection of nitrogen mustard into the pleural space or by ligation of the thoracic duct.

FURTHER READING

Fraser R G, Pare J A P 1979 Diagnosis of diseases of the chest. 2nd edn. Saunders, Philadelphia.

Harley H R S 1979 Malignant pleural effusions and their treatment by intercostal talc pleurodesis. British Journal of Diseases of the Chest 73:173

23

Pneumothorax ⎧ traumatic
⎨ spontaneous ⎧ Apices, young, normal lung
⎩ (subpleural bullae) ⎨ Apices too. Older, emphysematous
⎩ Rare aron bron
— staph lung abscess
— TB cavity rupture
— asthma M:F
— bronchial Ca 5:1
— fibrosing alveolitis

Spontaneous pneumothorax

DEFINITION

The presence of air in the pleural space is called pneumothorax. The term 'spontaneous pneumothorax' is used when pneumothorax occurs unexpectedly and is secondary to disease of the lungs or pleura. Pneumothorax due to rib fractures, crushed chest injuries or penetrating wounds is called traumatic pneumothorax.

EPIDEMIOLOGY

Spontaneous pneumothorax can occur at any age but is most common in apparently healthy people aged 20 to 40. Men are affected five times more often than women and the annual incidence in young men is 40 per 100 000. The other common age for pneumothorax is between 50 and 60 years where it occurs predominantly in men with chronic bronchitis and emphysema.

AETIOLOGY

Rupture of subpleural emphysematous bullae.
This is the main cause of pneumothorax in both healthy young people and in older people. In the first group, small thin-walled cysts are present in the apex of the lung and the remainder of the lung is normal. The factors responsible for these apical cysts are not known, but their development may be related to the relatively reduced perfusion and the increased mechanical stresses which occur at the apex of the lung. The mechanical stresses are influenced by gravity and are greater in lungs with large vertical dimensions, which may explain the prevalence of pneumothorax in tall, thin individuals. Alternatively the apical cysts may be a congenital anomaly. In contrast, in older patients, in addition to apical bullae there is often

evidence of widespread emphysema, and this is usually accompanied by chronic bronchitis.

Uncommon causes

Pneumothorax is occasionally caused by a staphylococcal lung abscess or a tuberculous cavity rupturing into the pleural space. This results in a pyopneumothorax if pus as well as air enters the pleural space. Pneumothorax is a rare complication of asthma, bronchial carcinoma and fibrosing alveolitis.

PATHOGENESIS

In health the parietal and visceral pleura are separated by a potential space, and the pressure in this space, the intrapleural pressure, is subatmospheric. If a hole develops in the visceral pleura, air is drawn from the lung into the pleural space by the subatmospheric intrapleural pressure. Air may also enter the pleural space through a hole in the parietal pleura if the hole extends through the layers of the chest wall. This may occur accidentally during aspiration of a pleural effusion. Air in the pleural space allows the lung to recoil towards the hilum and may cause displacement of the mediastinum to the opposite side.

Pneumothorax may be classified according to the sequence of events which follows the breach in the pleura.

Closed pneumothorax. The hole in the pleura closes after a short interval; the air in the pleural space is absorbed and the lung re-expands.

Open pneumothorax. In an open pneumothorax the communication between the lung and the pleural space remains patent and air moves in and out of the pleural space during respiration. This prevents re-expansion of the lung. Occasionally a communication develops between a bronchus and the pleural space. This is called a *bronchopleural fistula* and in these cases the intrapleural pressure may be equal to atmospheric pressure.

Tension pneumothorax. Occasionally the hole in the pleura acts as a valve so that air enters the pleural space during inspiration but cannot escape during expiration. There is progressive increase in the intrapleural pressure which rises above atmospheric pressure so that the lung collapses and the mediastinum is increasingly displaced to the opposite side, causing compression of the great vessels and the opposite lung. If tension pneumothorax is not treated immediately, the patient may die from hypoxaemia and circulatory collapse.

FUNCTIONAL ABNORMALITY

The functional effects and the clinical features are determined mainly by the size of the pneumothorax and the patient's pulmonary function. The latter may be impaired by the presence of pre-existing respiratory diseases, especially chronic bronchitis and emphysema.

Pneumothorax causes reduction in lung volumes and diffusing capacity, and there may be transient hypoxaemia due to shunting of blood through the collapsed lung.

CLINICAL FEATURES

Onset. The onset is usually sudden with pleuritic pain and breathlessness.

Pleuritic pain. The pain is often severe and is unilateral. Pain is sometimes referred to the shoulder tip on the affected side as a result of irritation of the diaphragmatic pleura. In 10 per cent of patients pain is absent.

Breathlessness. This is common when pneumothorax occurs in patients with poor pulmonary function due to emphysema. In contrast, in healthy young patients even a large pneumothorax may not cause breathlessness.

Persistent irritating cough is occasionally the presenting symptom. Sometimes the patient complains of a clicking sound over the left side of the lower chest. This occurs with a shallow left pneumothorax and may be due to movement of an intrapleural pocket of air by the cardiac pulsation.

There may be symptoms of the disease which has given rise to the pneumothorax, and the patient should always be asked about recent chest injury because of the possibility that the pneumothorax is traumatic in origin.

Physical examination. Dyspnoea, central cyanosis and tachycardia are present if the pneumothorax is large or if the patient has severe chronic bronchitis and emphysema. The signs of air in the pleural space are not obvious if the pneumothorax is small. A large pneumothorax may cause diminished chest movement, hyperresonant percussion note, and diminished or absent breath sounds on the affected side and mediastinal displacement to the opposite side.

INVESTIGATIONS

Chest radiograph. This shows a clearly defined lung edge with absence of lung markings between the lung and the chest wall

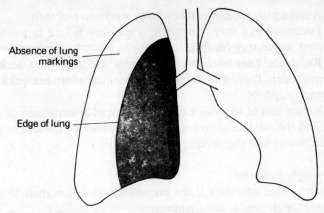

Absence of lung markings

Edge of lung

Fig. 39 Pneumothorax.

(Fig. 39). The pneumothorax may be localized if part of the pleura remains in contact with the chest wall because of previous adhesions. Mediastinal displacement is present if the pneumothorax is large, and the costophrenic angle may be obliterated by a small collection of serous fluid or blood. The chest radiograph should be examined for fractured ribs.

A small pneumothorax may be missed if it is not specifically looked for, and sometimes it is only seen in a radiograph taken in full expiration.

It is helpful to grade the size of a pneumothorax in terms of the percentage of the hemithorax occupied by the pneumothorax, i.e. a 75 per cent pneumothorax is one occupying 75 per cent of the hemithorax.

DIFFERENTIAL DIAGNOSIS

A chest radiograph will differentiate pneumothorax from *pneumonia*, *pulmonary infarction*, and *myocardial infarction*. *Large emphysematous bullae* (p. 140) resemble a localized pneumothorax in the radiograph. Recent chest pain or sudden increase in breathlessness is in favour of pneumothorax. Pleurodynia causes pleuritic pain but is accompanied by localized intercostal tenderness and fever.

TREATMENT

The management of spontaneous pneumothorax requires an appreciation of the following facts:

1. Pneumothorax is a potentially serious condition because of the complications.

2. A large pneumothorax takes many weeks to reabsorb.

3. Pneumothorax may precipitate respiratory failure in patients with poor respiratory function.

4. Recurrent pneumothorax is common and may have serious consequences in those who cannot obtain medical assistance quickly, e.g. seamen, pilots.

The main aim of treatment is to obtain rapid re-expansion of the lung, and the method of treatment is determined by the size of the pneumothorax and the severity of the dyspnoea.

Conservative treatment

No treatment is necessary if the pneumothorax is less than 30 per cent and the patient is not dyspnoeic.

Generally it is wise to admit the patient to hospital unless he lives close to medical assistance which can be obtained immediately if he becomes acutely dyspnoeic. The patient must be kept under observation until the lung has re-expanded and should avoid strenuous activity for several weeks.

Insertion of an intercostal catheter

This is indicated if the pneumothorax is causing breathlessness or if it is more than 30 per cent in size. The catheter is inserted through the second intercostal space in the midclavicular line. In young women, it is preferable to use the fifth intercostal space in the axilla for cosmetic reasons. A self retaining catheter, such as a Malecot catheter, is introduced into the pleural space, with the aid of a trochar and cannula. An alternative to this is a plastic catheter which is supplied with its own introducer. Care must be taken to avoid sudden uncontrolled deep penetration of the chest wall which may damage the underlying lung and vessels. The intrapleural catheter is connected to an underwater seal drainage system which allows air to leave the pleural space but prevents it from re-entering. The catheter is connected to the longer arm of the glass tubing. (Fig. 40).

The water level in the glass tube fluctuates with the changes in intrapleural pressure during inspiration and expiration. If the 'tube stops swinging', either the lung is fully expanded or the tube is blocked. If the tube is blocked it is usually necessary to insert a new catheter in a fresh site. After the lung is fully expanded the catheter is left in situ for 48 hours to encourage adhesions to develop between the layers of the pleura because this may prevent recurrence. Usually the catheter is removed 4 to 5 days after insertion and the patient can return to work the following week.

An alternative to underwater seal drainage is a small valve which may be attached to the end of the intercostal catheter thus allowing

Rx.
- Conservative (if <30%, not dyspnoeic)
- Catheter, O₂,
  ABs if inf⁷.
- pleurodesis ← if bilateral
  same side x 3
- thoracotomy.

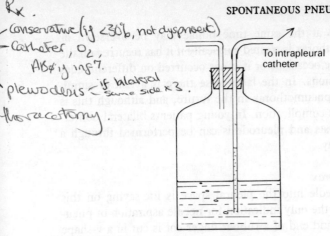

To intrapleural
catheter

Fig. 40 Underwater seal drainage system.

the patient to be ambulant. Oxygen is given if the patient is breathless and antibiotics are necessary if there is pulmonary infection.

TREATMENT OF COMPLICATIONS

Chronic pneumothorax
Failure of the lung to re-expand after treatment with an intercostal catheter for several days may be due to pulmonary collapse from retained secretions or due to a persistent air leak or a bronchopleural fistula. Collapse is treated by bronchoscopy and aspiration of secretions. A persistent air leak or a bronchopleural fistula are indications for thoracotomy; the site of the air leak or fistula is identified and is locally resected.

Recurrent pneumothorax
Recurrence occurs in 30 per cent of patients after the initial attack, and thereafter the recurrence rate increases if the patient is treated conservatively. There is disagreement about the best method of treatment. Insertion of an intercostal catheter may prevent further recurrence by causing pleural adhesions. Irritants introduced into the pleural space may also cause pleurodesis; silver nitrate solution, iodized talc and camphor in oil are used for this purpose, but the success rate is variable.

Alternatively, thoracotomy is carried out and the subpleural bullae responsible for the pneumothorax are oversewn or resected and the parietal pleura is abraded to promote adhesions. Parietal pleurectomy prevents recurrence but this involves a major operation. The parietal pleura is stripped from the chest wall and upper mediastinum and at the same time bullae may be oversewn or resected. Pneumothorax is treated surgically if it has recurred on the same side on three occasions or if it has occurred on different sides on separate occasions. In the latter case there is a risk of simultaneous bilateral pneumothorax in the future, and although this is rare it is a serious complication. In young patients bilateral obliteration of apical cysts and pleurodesis can be performed through a median sternotomy.

Tension pneumothorax

Insertion of a needle into the pleural space is life-saving on this emergency and is the only indication for needle aspiration of pneumothorax. The blind end of a rubber finger cot is cut in a v-shape and the open end is tied around the end of the needle to act as a valve. The needle should be replaced by an intercostal catheter as soon as possible.

Haemopneumothorax

Rupture of pleural adhesions may cause massive intrapleural haemorrhage. This is a rare complication and is treated by transfusion and thoracotomy.

Pyopneumothorax

The pus is drained through an intercostal catheter and antibiotics are given. Sometimes rib resection is necessary to achieve adequate drainage of pus.

Subcutaneous emphysema, mediastinal emphysema

These are rare complications of spontaneous pneumothorax and usually accompany traumatic pneumothorax.

FURTHER READING

Crompton G K 1982 Spontaneous pneumothorax. Hospital Update March: 251
Horne N W 1966 Spontaneous pneumothorax: diagnosis and management. British Medical Journal i: 281
Lichter I, Gwynne J F 1971 Spontaneous pneumothorax in young subjects, a clinical and pathological study. Thorax 26: 409
Ruckley C V, McCormack R J M 1966 The management of spontaneous pneumothorax. Thorax 21: 139
Watts R E, Bennett D J, Horton D A, Wright J S 1970 Spontaneous pneumothorax, a rational approach to treatment. Medical Journal of Australia 1: 538
West J B 1971 Distribution of mechanical stress in the lung, a possible factor in the localisation of pulmonary disease. Lancet i: 839

24

Rare disorders

Cystic fibrosis

This hereditary disorder is transmitted in a recessive manner and affects 1 baby per 2500 live births. The basic abnormality is poorly understood but it appears that production of abnormal mucus is responsible for the main features of the disease. The newborn with cystic fibrosis may present with acute intestinal obstruction due to meconium ileus. In infancy, failure to thrive and steatorrhoea occur as a result of disturbance of pancreatic function. In the older child the abnormal mucus in the respiratory tract predisposes to recurrent respiratory infections. Staphylococcal pneumonia and infections with *Pseudomonas* and *H. influenzae* are common. The child usually has persistent loose cough and finger clubbing; in 10 per cent of cases nasal polypi are present.

Children with cystic fibrosis excrete excessive amounts of salt in their sweat, and the most useful test for diagnosis is the sweat test. The diagnosis is confirmed if the sweat sodium exceeds 70 mEq/l.

Treatment includes prophylactic chemotherapy with flucloxacillin, pancreatic enzyme supplements, regular physiotherapy with aerosol inhalations, avoidance of cross infection and prompt treatment of acute infections. About 80 per cent of children now survive to adult life. Pseudomonas becomes the predominant pathogen in adults. Respiratory failure and cor pulmonale eventually supervene in all but the mildest cases.

Collagen disorders

In teaching hospitals collagen disorders are oft sought but seldom found, simply because they are rare. It is a sobering thought that even in Western countries more people die from undiagnosed tuberculosis than from collagen disorders.

Collagen disorders produce a variety of reactions in the respiratory system. The respiratory tract may be the only site of disease but often other systems are involved. The diagnosis of a collagen disorder is usually suggested by the presence of systemic lesions, positive anti-nuclear factor and a very high ESR. Biopsy of affected tissue is used to confirm the diagnosis, renal biopsy providing a guide to prognosis. This is usually poor in systemic sclerosis and polyarteritis nodosa but treatment with corticosteroids prolongs survival in systemic lupus erythematosus.

Rheumatoid arthritis

The respiratory manifestations of rheumatoid arthritis are more common in males than females.

Pleural effusion (p. 234) is the commonest respiratory manifestation and is usually unilateral. The pleural fluid is an exudate and characteristically has a low glucose content and contains rheumatoid factor. The effusion usually resolves after repeated aspiration.

Fibrosing alveolitis (p. 223) occurs in 5 per cent of patients with rheumatoid arthritis. It cannot be differentiated clinically from fibrosing alveolitis associated with other diseases, apart from the presence of rheumatoid arthritis. It does not usually respond to corticosteroids.

Rheumatoid nodules (p. 178) rarely cause symptoms, and are usually first detected as single or multiple rounded opacities in the chest radiograph. The nodules may cavitate. Rheumatoid nodules do not require treatment.

Caplan's syndrome (p. 214) comprises rheumatoid arthritis, coal workers' pneumoconiosis and rheumatoid nodules in the lung. The nodules occur in the periphery of the lung and sometimes they appear before the arthritis.

Rheumatoid laryngitis due to rheumatoid involvement of the cricoarytenoid joints causes hoarseness, stridor and sometimes complete laryngeal obstruction.

Obliterative bronchiolitis with consequent small airways obstruction is sometimes associated with rheumatoid arthritis and does not respond to corticosteroids.

Systemic lupus erythematosus

The respiratory system is one of the many systems which may be involved by this systemic disorder. Systemic lupus erythematosus mainly occurs in young or middle-aged females. The diagnosis is usually confirmed by finding LE cells, ANF or anti-DNA antibodies in the blood.

Pleurisy and pleural effusion (p. 234) are not uncommon in systemic lupus erythematosus; the pleural fluid is an exudate and may contain LE cells and ANF.

Pneumonia in systemic lupus erythematosus may be due to lung involvement by the disease itself or to bacterial infection.

Fibrosing alveolitis is a rare manifestation of systemic lupus erythematosus.

Systemic sclerosis
This disorder mainly occurs in young or middle-aged females. Respiratory involvement is usually accompanied by typical shiny, sclerotic skin changes and lesions in the oesophagus, joints and kidney. The diagnosis is confirmed by biopsy of affected tissues.

Fibrosing alveolitis (p. 224) causes dyspnoea and a restrictive ventilatory defect, sometimes without radiographic evidence of fibrosis.

Pneumonia may occur as a result of spillover if the oesophagus is involved by scleroderma.

Polyarteritis nodosa
The respiratory system is involved in about 30 per cent of patients with polyarteritis nodosa. The respiratory lesions of polyarteritis nodosa are accompanied by blood eosinophilia and form part of the spectrum of pulmonary eosinophilia. Involvement of the kidneys, central nervous system, heart, alimentary tract, joints and skin is common.

Asthma is sometimes the first manifestation of polyarteritis nodosa. The asthma is chronic and severe, and is characterized by very high eosinophil counts.

Pneumonia and *necrotic pulmonary lesions* due to polyarteritis nodosa cause cough and haemoptysis.

Corticosteroids help the asthma and may help the other pulmonary manifestations.

Pulmonary eosinophilia
Pulmonary eosinophilia is the name given to a group of disorders characterized by recurrent pulmonary infiltrations, cough, wheeze, fever and eosinophilia of the peripheral blood. Occasionally the patient coughs up yellowish plugs of mucus which contain eosinophils. The chest radiograph shows localized patchy shadowing which disappears after a few weeks or months only to reappear shortly after in a different part of the lung. The commonest cause of pulmonary eosinophilia is hypersensitivity to *A. fumigatus*—allergic bronchopulmonary aspergillosis (p. 119). Other causes include allergic reactions to parasitic worms such as *Ascaris lumbricoides* or filaria, or to drugs such as penicillin, aspirin and nitrofurantoin. Frequently the symptoms and pulmonary infiltrations resolve spontaneously, but it may be necessary to give corticosteroids. *Polyarteritis nodosa* may manifest as pulmonary eosinophilia.

Idiopathic pulmonary haemosiderosis

Idiopathic pulmonary haemosiderosis is a disorder of unknown aetiology in which recurrent intrapulmonary haemorrhage results in deposition of haemosiderin within the lungs, causing variable degrees of interstitial fibrosis. The disease usually starts in childhood and the main features are recurrent haemoptysis and iron deficiency anaemia. The severity of the pulmonary haemorrhage is variable and ranges from slight bloodstaining of the sputum in the early stages of the disease to massive haemoptysis which may be fatal. Symptoms of anaemia include tiredness and pallor, and blood examination shows hypochromic anaemia, reticulocytosis and low serum iron. The sputum may contain haemosiderin containing macrophages but this finding is not diagnostic since it may occur in other diseases which cause pulmonary haemorrhage. The chest radiograph shows transient pulmonary opacities after haemorrhagic episodes and in the later stages of the disease there may be persistent military mottling. Exacerbations and remissions are common. During exacerbations, treatment with corticosteroids in high doses may be beneficial but long-term treatment is of doubtful value. The anaemia is treated with iron and if necessary transfusion. The outcome is extremely variable but many patients die within five years.

Goodpasture's syndrome

Goodpasture's syndrome is characterized by pulmonary haemorrhage and glomerulonephritis, and is probably an immune disorder related to polyarteritis nodosa and idiopathic pulmonary haemosiderosis. It is commonest in young males and the patient usually presents with recurrent haemoptysis which is followed within a few weeks or months by proteinuria, haematuria and progressive renal failure. Anti-glomerular basement membrane antibody is found in the serum. Renal biopsy will confirm the presence of glomerulonephritis. Corticosteroids, immunosuppresives and plasmapheresis may sometimes be beneficial but usually the disease is fatal.

Wegener's granulomatosis

Wegener's granulomatosis is a syndrome of unknown aetiology characterized by necrotizing granulomatous lesions of the respiratory tract, generalized focal necrotizing vasculitis and necrotizing glomerulitis. Wegener's granulomatosis mainly occurs in middle-aged adults. Granulomas commonly involve the nose and para-nasal sinuses, producing nasal obstruction, purulent nasal discharge and epistaxis. Granulomas in the lung cause persistent cough, haemoptysis and pleuritic pain. The chest radiograph shows large dense opacities which may cavitate. Constitutional symptoms include malaise, weight loss and fever. Proteinuria and haematuria indicate renal involvement. Death from uraemia used to occur within six months but more recently the use of high-dose prednisolone with cyclophosphamide or azathioprine has improved the prognosis.

Shock lung

This condition, sometimes called 'adult respiratory distress syndrome' or 'post-traumatic pulmonary insufficiency', is characterised by increasing breathlessness and cough, crepitations, alveolar infiltrates and progressive hypoxaemia. It can be a sequel to haemorrhagic or septic shock, trauma, viral pneumonia, aspiration of gastric contents or haemorrhagic pancreatitis. Treatment usually involves morphine, diuretics, oxygen, mechanical ventilation ± PEEP, digoxin and removal or correction of the precipitating factor.

FURTHER READING

Anderson C, Goodchild M 1976 Cystic fibrosis: manual of diagnosis and treatment. Blackwell, Oxford

Crofton J, Douglas A 1981 Respiratory diseases. 3rd edn. Blackwell, Oxford.

Grant I W B 1979 Drug-induced diseases: drug induced respiratory disease. British Medical Journal i: 1070

Grant I W B 1982 Bronchopulmonary eosinophilia. Hospital Update April: 491

Hodson M, Norman A P, Batten J C 1983 Cystic fibrosis. Balliere Tindall, London

Middleton W G, Paterson J C, Grant I W B, Douglas A C 1977 Asthmatic pulmonary eosinophilia. A review of 65 cases. British Journal of Diseases of the Chest 71: 115

Morgan P G M, Turner-Warwick M 1981 Pulmonary haemosiderosis and pulmonary haemorrhage. British Journal of Diseases of the Chest 75:225

Murray J F 1980 Adult respiratory distress syndrome. In: Flenley D C (ed) Recent advances in respiratory medicine. Livingstone, 67, Edinburgh pleura and pleuritic pain. The chest radiograph shows large dense opacities which may cavitate. Constitutional symptoms include malaise, weight loss and fever. Pneumonia and haematuria indicate renal involvement. Death from vasculitis used to occur within six months, but more recently the use of high-dose prednisolone with cyclophosphamide or azathioprine has improved the prognosis.

Shock lung

This condition, sometimes called 'adult respiratory distress syndrome' or 'post-traumatic pulmonary insufficiency', is characterised by increasing breathlessness and cough, frequently absolute intolerance and progressive hypoxaemia. It can be a sequel to haemorrhagic or septic shock, trauma, viral pneumonia, aspiration of gastric contents or haemorrhagic pancreatitis. Treatment usually involves prolonged artificial oxygen, mechanical ventilation and PEEP, and removal or correction of the precipitating factor.

FURTHER READING

Crofton J, Douglas A 1981 Respiratory diseases, 3rd ed. Blackwell, Oxford
Flenley D C 1990 Respiratory medicine, 2nd ed. Baillière Tindall, London
Seaton A, Seaton D, Leitch A G 1989 Crofton and Douglas's respiratory diseases, 4th ed. Blackwell, Oxford
Macfarlane J T 1986 Recent advances in community-acquired pneumonia. In: Gould D, Lenfant C (eds) Advances in respiratory medicine. Churchill, Edinburgh

Index